KU-450-307

# Clinic Handbook
# of Women's Health

**Diana Hamilton-Fairley**
*Consultant Obstetrician and Gynaecologist,
Guy's and St Thomas' Hospitals NHS Trust,
London, UK*

**Debra Holloway**
*Consultant Gynaecology Nurse, Guy's and
St Thomas' Hospitals NHS Trust,
London, UK*

**Gabriel Taylor**
*Gynaecology Service Manager, Guy's and
St Thomas' Hospitals NHS Trust,
London, UK*

© BIOS Scientific Publishers Limited, 2003

First published in 2003

All rights reserved. No part of this book may be reproduced or transmitted, in any form or by any means, without permission.

A CIP catalogue record for this book is available from the British Library.

ISBN 1 85996 098 7

BIOS Scientific Publishers Ltd
9 Newtec Place, Magdalen Road, Oxford OX4 1RE, UK
Tel. +44 (0)1865 726286. Fax +44 (0)1865 246823
World Wide Web home page: http: //www.bios.co.uk/

*Important Note from the Publisher*
The information contained within this book was obtained by BIOS Scientific Publishers Ltd from sources believed by us to be reliable. However, while every effort has been made to ensure its accuracy, no responsibility for loss or injury whatsoever occasioned to any person acting or refraining from action as a result of information contained herein can be accepted by the authors or publishers.

The reader should remember that medicine is a constantly evolving science and while the authors and publishers have ensured that all dosages, applications and practices are based on current indications, there may be specific practices which differ between communities. You should always follow the guidelines laid down by the manufacturers of specific products and the relevant authorities in the country in which you are practising.

Production Editor: Andrea Bosher.
Typeset by Saxon Graphics Ltd, Derby, UK.
Printed by TJ International, Padstow, UK.

University of Nottingham
at Derby Library

1003178639 T

# Contents

## Section 1  Planning and management of outpatients

## Section 2  Clinical gynaecological management of outpatients

## Section 3  Roles and training of outpatients staff

# Abbreviations

| | |
|---|---|
| AFP | alphafetoprotein |
| APS | antiphospholipid syndrome |
| BMI | body mass index |
| BSO | bilateral salpingo-oophorectomy |
| CIN | cervical intaepithelial neoplasia |
| COCP | combined oral contraceptive pill |
| CVD | cardiovascular disease |
| DNA | did not attend |
| DVT | deep vein thrombosis |
| E2 | estradiol |
| ECG | electrocardiogram |
| EPR | electronic patient record |
| FBC | full blood count |
| FSH | follicle stimulating hormone |
| GnRH | gonadotrophin releasing hormone |
| GOPD | gynaecology outpatients department |
| GP | general practitioner |
| GU | genito-urinary |
| HCG | human chorionic gonadotrophin |
| HFEA | human fertilization and embryology authority |
| HH | hypogoadotrophic hypogonadism |
| HRT | hormone replacement therapy |
| HSG | hysterosalpingogram |
| HVS | high vaginal swab |
| HyCoSy | hysterocontrastsalpingography |
| ICSO | intracytoplasmic sperm injection |
| IMB | intermenstural bleeding |
| ISC | intermittent self catheterization |
| IU/L | international unit per litre |
| IUCD | intrauterine contraceptive device |
| IUI | intrauterine insemination |
| IUS | intrauterine system |
| IVF | in-vitro fertilization |
| LH | luteinising hormone |
| LHRH | luteinising hormone releasing hormone |
| MC&S | microscopy, culture and sensitivity |
| MRI | magnetic resonance imaging |
| MS | multiple sclerosis |

| MSU | mid-stream urine |
| NHSCSP | National Health Service cervical screening programme |
| NSAID | non-steroidal anti-inflammatory drugs |
| PCB | post-coital bleeding |
| PCOS | polysystic ovary syndrome |
| PCR | polymerase chain reaction |
| PE | pulmonary embolus |
| PGD | preimplantation genetic diagnosis |
| PID | pelvic inflammatory disease |
| PMB | postmenopausal bleeding |
| POF | premature ovarian failure |
| POP | progesterone only pill |
| PRL | prolactin |
| RM | recurrent miscarriage |
| SC-J | squamo-columnar junction |
| SERM | selective estrogen receptor modulators |
| T | testosterone |
| T4 | thyroxine |
| TAH | total abdominal hysterectomy |
| TFT | thyroid function test |
| TSH | thyroid stimulating hormone |
| UTI | urinary tract infection |

# Contributors

**Diana Hamilton-Fairley MD FRCOG**
Consultant Obstetrician and
Gynaecologist,
Guy's and St. Thomas' Hospitals, NHS
Trust, London, UK

**Debra Holloway**
Consultant Gynaecology Nurse, Guy's and
St. Thomas' Hospitals, NHS Trust,
London, UK

**Sonya Hoy**
Specialist Nurse, Gynaecological
Oncology, St. Thomas' Hospital, London,
UK

**Aggie Johkan**
Nurse Practioner, Colposcopy, Guy's
Hospital, London, UK

**Ellie Stewart**
Sister, Department of Urology, Guy's
Hospital, London, UK

**Gabriel Taylor**
Gynaecology Service Manager, Guy's and
St. Thomas' Hospitals, NHS Trust,
London, UK

# Preface

Gynaecology outpatients are a complex clinical area that requires team working across many professional and non-professional groups. We have combined as a team of a consultant gynaecologist, consultant nurse and service manager to write this book in an attempt to cover the processes that have to take place in order for a patient to be seen and treated appropriately. It includes chapters on the organization and problems undertaken by the clerical and secretarial staff often behind the scenes. Patients and clinicians are often unaware of the enormous number of steps required from receipt of a referral letter to the successful completion of the patient episode that are dependent on clerical staff. This book aims to highlight those processes and the coordination and systems needed to make the flow efficient and seamless.

The clinical section is not designed as a textbook of gynaecological conditions and assumes a reasonable knowledge of gynaecology in its readership. The aim is to provide guidelines and flow charts for the management of common conditions seen in outpatients. Some of the women may never need admission and increasingly can be managed entirely as outpatients. Recent advances in technology allow many more investigations to be carried out in the outpatient clinic setting and this book concentrates on the setting up and running of one-stop clinics, rapid access clinics and nurse-led clinics. The role of the nurse is changing considerably and this book highlights areas that allow nurses to expand their role and take full clinical responsibility for a case load.

The book is therefore designed for gynaecology outpatient managers, nurses, specialist registrars and newly appointed consultants. The layout is deliberately in short chapters with flow charts, boxes and tables for easy and quick reference.

We would like to thank all our contributors. The greatest thanks, though, goes to all the hard work of the clerical, secretarial and administrative staff in the McNair Centre at Guy's Hospital who have been so instrumental in setting up our outpatient clinics and the constant development and expansion of the services we provide.

# Planning and Management of Outpatients

# 1 | Planning and Management of Outpatients

## Managing referral letters

The ideal management process for referral letters received by a gynaecology outpatients department is shown in *Figure 1.1*. The whole process relies on a teamwork approach by clinic staff, GPs, clerks and the patients. The process can be refined if simple measures are in place.

These include:

- a definition and understanding of the role played by each of the team members;
- an understanding of any local or national targets and how the department is to achieve these;
- the use of proformas/protocols for referral direct from the GP into outpatient clinics;
- the use of fax/email for referral letters;
- a protocol for vetting of referral letters internally;
- a protocol for investigations needed prior to the clinic appointment;
- clear guidelines for dealing with letters that are asking for advice or clarification.

## Processing of referral letters

The referral process starts when the patient visits her GP with a problem/condition that needs advice/treatment from a gynaecologist.

Once the patient has been referred for consultation, treatment or advice a letter is generated. These letters are then sent to a central point within the hospital (Patient Registration) by post, fax or email. The referrals are sorted by a clerk and given a hospital number and then sent to gynaecology outpatients.

Once in gynaecology outpatients the letters are:

- date stamped;
- graded as part of the vetting system into: routine, soon, urgent, and 2 week cancer waits (all letters that state urgent and/or 2 week cancer waits should be put to one side to be vetted to a special rapid access clinic and appointments made immediately);
- vetted to the most appropriate clinic based on presenting complaint.

Using a system where conditions are vetted to a clinic rather than a named consultant, means that patients are seen by the most appropriate health care professional.

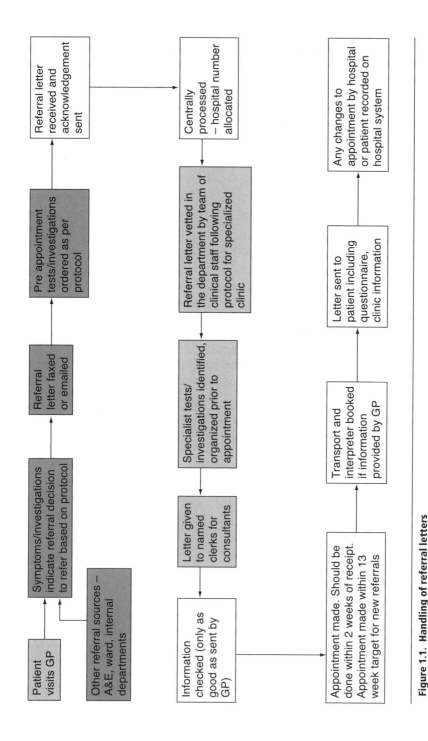

**Figure 1.1. Handling of referral letters**

Once the patient has been given a hospital number an appointment can be made. Most systems will generate a standard letter and the clerk can supplement this with pre-written information sheets or questionnaires for specific clinics.

This process should enable letters to be sorted into queries/advice that can be allocated to the most appropriate person. The vetting process should also be used to highlight extra information that the GP has supplied in relation to transport requests, interpreters and gender preference of the health care professional.

| Box 1.1 | Potential problems with the referral process |
|---|---|

- Lost letters
- Illegible letters
- Wrong patient information
- Tests not identified prior to appointment
- Letters vetted to wrong clinic
- No transport/interpreters booked – not highlighted by GP/missed on referral letter

## Responsibility for the process

As part of the vetting process each department should calculate a monthly waiting time for each consultant clinic. This, when used in conjunction with the presenting condition, will ensure that patients are seen within the national targets. Once vetted the letters should be entered onto a database to enable any future queries in relation to lost/mislaid letters to be dealt with. The named clerk for each consultant clinic will be responsible for making the appointments (*Box 1. 2*). Any patient information/leaflets, questionnaires and investigation requests will be included with the outpatient letter.

| Box 1.2 | Responsibilty of the team in the referral process |
|---|---|

| Process | Responsibility |
|---|---|
| Receipt/date | Patient Registration/Supervisors/Clerks/Secretaries |
| Vetting/grading/diagnostic requests | Consultant/ SpR / Nurse Practitioner |
| Data-base | Clerk/Secretary |
| Appointment/patient transport /interpreters | Supervisors/Clerks |
| Information leaflets | Supervisors/Clerks/Nurses |
| Notes | Medical records/Clerks |
| Notes preparation | Supervisors/Clerks/Nursing staff |
| Reception | Supervisors/Clerks |
| Follow-up appointments | Consultant team/Nurses/Clerks |
| DNAs – what to do? | Consultant team/Nurses/Clerks |

## Diagnostic management pre-appointment

The letters all need to be read by a senior clinician, doctor or nurse, the presenting complaint and any tests the GP has organized noted. The clinician vetting the letters should, by using local guidelines, request any further investigations that need to be organized prior to the clinic appointment. These can range from blood tests to scans and should be recorded on the referral letter so that the clinic clerk can check the test dates are organized prior to making the appointment. The clerk should include any test forms/appointments in the letter. In this way the patient should have had all the relevant tests needed to aid the clinical diagnosis and management of her condition prior to the first appointment.

## Information for patients

Information sent to patients should be:

- relevant;
- current.

Where appropriate it should be available in a form that is:

- user friendly;
- translated into various languages appropriate for the local community.

All information/instructions that are relevant for the first appointment should be included with the appointment letter, with clear instructions enabling the patient's journey to the clinic to be as simple as possible. All information/guidelines sent should be revised on a regular basis to allow for national and local updates to be incorporated.

Any changes that are made to this process and/or within each clinic must be communicated to the whole team. Any verbal or written information relayed to patients via front line staff should be uniform to avoid confusion for that patient.

# Management of clinic appointments

The efficient running of a clinic depends on the way that it is structured. The Royal College of Obstetricians and Gynaecologists has previously issued guidance concerning the timing of outpatient's appointments. It has suggested that new gynaecological outpatient referrals require 20 minutes and review (follow-up) cases 10 minutes. This is based on a traditional view that new patients require longer appointments than follow-up patients. However, as gynaecology outpatients are changing and specialist/one-stop clinics are being introduced this view needs to be re-examined (*Box 1.3*).

| Box 1.3 | Factors to consider in development of a clinic profile |
| --- | --- |

- Number of medical staff available
- Type of clinic
- Experience of available staff
- Number of nursing staff
- Number of nurse practitioners or specialist nurses
- Supervision and teaching of postgraduate trainees
- Undergraduate teaching
- Case-mix
- Associated procedure
- Organization of subsequent care

More patients are being treated conservatively and their follow-up visits often take longer than the first visit. This may occur for a number of reasons:

- patients want and deserve far more information about their condition and the proposed treatment;
- the patient has obtained a great deal of information that has increased her anxieties and requires answers to all that have been raised;
- a full review of the patient's condition is indicated;
- the treatment was not effective and requires review;
- patients needing interpreters or with special needs will need to have a longer consultation.

The following additional factors are likely to be contributing to changes in outpatient workload:

- fewer and less experienced junior staff;
- altered training targets for postgraduate trainees;
- patient's expectations;
- explicit clinical standards and use of guidelines;
- increasing access by patients to information;
- increased need for informed discussion, informed consent and counselling;
- development of special interest and sub-specialist clinics;
- pressure to achieve waiting times for appointments as outlined in the National Plan.

Each department will need to examine the following factors to determine the number of women who can be seen in an outpatient session:

- number of medical staff available;
- type of clinic;
- experience of available staff;
- number of nursing staff;
- number of nurse practitioners or specialist nurses;
- supervision and teaching of postgraduate trainees;
- undergraduate teaching;
- case-mix;
- associated procedure;
- organization of subsequent care.

It is essential that time is allowed for:

- each patient to be given adequate time for consultation (this is more than the time traditionally allocated);
- adequate documentation to be compiled within the notes;
- the electronic patient record (future) to be generated;

- the dictation of letters within the time-span of the clinic;
- the review any notes, results and queries from previous clinics.

There are, however, some specialist clinics where appointments will need to be longer. These are clinics treating conditions such as recurrent miscarriage where there will be counselling, or sub-fertility clinics where there are in fact two patients, the women and her partner. An appointment lasting 30 minutes is generally adequate for patients attending a one-stop clinic but only if there is an ultrasongrapher in the clinic to perform any necessary scans.

There is no standard way to write a clinic profile, this will depend upon the clinic type and a discussion with the clinic coordinator and consultant will be required. A team approach, involving consultants and trainees working within their own capabilities will determine the size of any specific clinic. The organization and mix of new and return patients will necessarily vary between individual clinics within a unit.

Clinic lists can be generated as one list for new and one for follow-ups with appointments for each time slot. The number of personnel available needs to be taken into account in this case. Alternatively, lists can be generated for the individual personnel in the clinic allowing the lists to be more flexible depending on the grade and experience of the clinician. This has the added advantage that the clinic can be effectively reduced if clinicians are away. If there is a nurse-led pre-clerking clinic alongside the general clinic, then space should be made on the consultants list for review of the patients and the consenting process. An example of a clinic profile is shown in *Box 1.4*.

The features to note in this profile are:

- The consultant sees more follow-ups than new patients. This has two advantages: (a) nearly all patients will see the consultant within three visits. This enables the results to be reviewed, a management plan made at senior level and all relevant information given to the patient by the consultant; (b) the junior staff are able to see the consultant and ask for advice and/or permission to place a patient on the waiting list more easily, as patients will come in and out of his/her office more often.
- The SHO is expected to see fewer patients.
- All post-operative follow-up patients are seen by the nurse practitioner, which frees up a large amount of medical time.
- The patients who are being admitted to an elective list are reviewed and consented by the consultant, allowing any last minute problems to be sorted out.
- The teaching session at the end is very valuable to all staff particularly junior medical staff and medical students.

Another initiative worth assessment is an evaluation of the role of initial clerking

| Box 1.4 | An example of a clinic profile | | | |
|---|---|---|---|---|
| Consultant | Registrar | SHO | NP | Pre clerking |
| New patient 09.00 | Return patient 09.00 | New patient 09.00 | Post operation FU 09.00 | 0900 |
| Return patient 09.20 | New patient 09.10 | New patient 09.20 | Post operation FU 09.20 | 0945 |
| Return patient Consent 09.30 | New patient 09.30 | Return patient 09.40 | New patient 09.40 | 10.30 |
| Return patient 09.30 | New patient 09.50 | New patient 10.00 | Post operation FU 10.00 | 11.15 |
| New patient Consent 10.00 | Return patient 10.10 | New patient 10.20 | Post operation FU 10.20 | 1200 |
| Return patient 10.20 | New patient 10.20 | New patient 10.40 | Post operation FU 10.40 | |
| New patient 10.30 | Return patient 10.30 | Return patient 11.10 | Post operation FU 11.00 | |
| Return patient Consent 10.50 | New patient 10.40 | New patient 11.30 | New patient 11.20 | |
| New patient 11.00 | Return patient 11.00 | | Return patient 11.40 | |
| Return patient 11.20 | New patient 11.20 | | Return patient 11.50 | |
| Return patient Consent 11.30 | Return patient 11.30 | | | |
| Return patient Consent 11.40 | | | | |
| **12.00. Review of cases with whole team** | | | | |

by nurses in special-interest clinics, following agreed protocols (hormone replacement therapy, infertility, urinary incontinence, family planning).

There is potential, with careful screening of referral letters, for arranging relevant blood tests and other investigations prior to first appointment in selected systemic categories. This may help to reduce the number of appointments necessary to complete initial assessment, reach a diagnosis and determine a treatment plan (menorrhagia, endocrine problems, infertility).

The outpatient department is the first contact most patients will have with the service. It is essential that this front-line service is adequately supported with clerical and secretarial staff as well as medical and nursing staff.

# Managing patients who fail to attend

Patients who fail to attend their clinic appointment can cause significant problems in relation to the correct management of clinic time. It is essential that the department has a policy to manage these cases for all clinics (*Figure 1.2*). The policy needs to be specific so those patients who have urgent and potentially cancerous conditions are not lost to the system. This will also ensure that patients who repeatedly do not attend (DNAs) are not given an excessive number of appointments that reduce the capacity of the clinics.

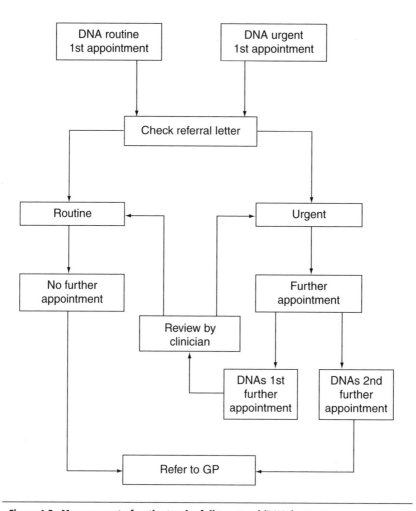

**Figure 1.2. Management of patients who fail to attend (DNAs)**

It is the responsibility of the clinic clerk to ensure that the notes of all patients who do not attend are brought to the attention of nursing or medical staff before the end of clinic. These notes should have been stamped DNA and include two options for the clinician (consultant, SpR 4/5, SpR 1-3 or nurse practitioner) to tick:

- send further appointment *or*
- no further appointment.

For patients who repeatedly do not attend but who telephone to make further appointments, the responsibility for this decision should not be left with the clerical staff. The patient should be informed that their hospital case notes will be obtained and the team that is caring for them will determine the need for an appointment.

## Guidelines for dealing with patients who have failed to attend

### Non-urgent first appointment

A standard letter from the hospital administration system should be sent to the GP, informing them that their patient did not attend and that a further appointment will not be offered without a second GP referral letter.

A standard letter should also be sent to the patient stating that if they still need to be seen they will need to be referred back by their GP.

### Urgent first appointment

If the patient had been vetted as an urgent patient then a letter should be sent to their GP as above, however, the letter should state that the patient has been given one further appointment.

A letter should be sent to the patient offering one further appointment and stating the need for them to attend this appointment. This letter should also include the contact details of the outpatients department if they have particular concerns or wish to change the date or time of the appointment.

If the clinician feels that there is a more urgent clinical need or the patient's details need checking, the patient and/or the GP will be telephoned

### DNA of the repeat appointment

If the patient DNAs a subsequent appointment then no further appointment should be made. A letter should be sent to both the patient and their GP informing them of the two DNAs and stating that the department is unable to offer any further appointments until the patient has seen their GP again.

## Follow-up appointments

### DNA of non-urgent follow-up appointment.

The nurse/doctor will review the previous visit to check if the patient is still in the routine category. If this proves to be the case then a letter will be sent to their GP informing him/her of their patient's DNA and the fact that a further appointment will not be offered.

A second letter can be sent to the patient stating that if they still need to be seen they will need to be referred back by their GP. The patient's care is then referred back to their GP.

If, however, on review the patient is re-classified as urgent then a subsequent appointment should be made.

### DNA of urgent follow-up appointment

A clinician will review the previous clinic visit to assess if the patient is still classified as urgent. If the patient is re-classified as routine then the management plan above can be followed. If they are still classified as urgent a letter should be sent to their GP to inform them of the patient's DNA. A letter should also be sent to the patient offering one further appointment

If the clinician feels that it would be of benefit then the patient and their GP should be telephoned, where possible, to confirm the urgent nature of the appointment.

## Communication with community services and patients

To ensure that there is an efficient gynaecology outpatient service the infrastructure needs to encompass an effective system of communication between the patient, primary care and the hospital.

The process starts when the patients visits her GP, health centre or Family Planning Service who then decides to refer on to secondary or tertiary care.

The referral letter should include the following information to aid rapid and accurate processing:

- patients demographic details including phone number and possibly email address;
- the presenting problem;
- previous relevant history;
- language problems;
- mobility problems.

This can be effectively communicated via a letter or using a proforma that is most commonly posted or in urgent cases faxed through to a central point within the department or hospital.

The technology now exists for the proforma, available via the PC, to be emailed direct to the outpatient clinic and for the patient to leave the doctor's surgery with an appointment (patient-agreed booking).

The use of proformas for 'target patients' who have suspected gynaecological cancers has speeded up the process. The use of the proforma for 'Target patients' enables the referral to be easily identified amongst the routine referral letters. However, the increasing use of proformas can increase the amount of paperwork the referrer has to fill in which acts as a disincentive for their use.

Once the referral letter has been received, processed and an appointment made a letter is normally generated by the hospital administration system. These letters will contain all the relevant information that the patient is likely to need prior to their appointment. This includes:

- the location of the hospital with details of local public transport;
- the location of the clinic (ideally with a map);
- the date and time of the appointment;
- the lead clinician's name/the name of the clinic (e.g. colposcopy);
- a contact number in case the patient needs to cancel or change their appointment;
- the length of time a patient may reasonably expect to be in the clinic.

If it is a speciality clinic, leaflets relevant to that clinic (e.g. one-stop, rapid access, implant, colposcopy) should be included along with a contact number for the Sister in outpatients in case the patients have any queries regarding their procedure.

After a patient has been seen it is usual to send a letter to their GP and/or the referrer if this is not the GP. This is dictated by the clinician at the end of clinic, typed by the consultant team secretary and sent out by post (see *Boxes 1.5* and *1.6*).

| Box 1.5 | Information for the patient |
| --- | --- |

**Letter for appointment**
Time and date
Name of clinic/consultant
Location of the clinic within the hospital
Time the patient should expect to spend in hospital
Contact number

**Enclosures**
Map with directions to clinic and transport/parking details
Information leaflets for specific clinics
Investigation forms with appointment dates (ultrasound) or instructions of how to get investigations performed (GP or hospital)

Increasingly, faxes and email are playing a role in this communication process. All letters should be faxed or mailed to a central point, which is usually Patient

Registration, so that there is no time delay whilst the letter goes round the department and in some cases the entire hospital.

Many departments now have an electronic patient record (EPR) that, if designed and used properly, will produce a letter generated from the consultation notes that can be sent to the GP/referrer without the need for dictation. This requires a great deal of commitment both financially and clinically to make sure the record makes sense and incorporates all the information needed for the finished letter. In the long-term there is hope that the hospital EPR will link directly with primary care computerized records so removing the need for paper in the whole process.

| Box 1.6 | Structured letter from clinic |
| --- | --- |

- Hospital Number for future reference
- Details of patient
- Presenting complaint
- Differential diagnosis
- Investigation and/or result
- Management options/plan
- Follow-up plan
- Free text

With increased pressure on outpatient services, patients are no longer routinely given a follow-up appointment with a consultant to obtain the results of tests or specimens. The development of nurse-led clinics and help-lines are being used more and more to replace junior doctors who traditionally saw the more routine patients as part of their role. A way of coordinating these results needs to be established so that the information is sent or communicated by phone or email to both the patients and their GP/referrer, together with any future management plans relevant to that patient.

Waiting times for appointments, both new and follow-up, are so great that the service provider needs to work and communicate more closely with the service user and listen to their needs. Patients are now seeking the "hands off" approach to medicine; a prime example being NHS direct. Use of this service continues to increase; patients now "surf the net" to find answers to their ailments and the availability of the treatment they want. It is probable that increasing use of specialty-based help-lines and email clinics may become part of clinical practice. However, there are issues surrounding confidentiality and clinical governance that must be addressed before electronic and non face-to-face consultations become routine.

## Equipping and designing outpatient clinics in gynaecology

The equipment and design of gynaecology outpatients will depend on the space available and the types of clinics that are to be undertaken.

General gynaecology clinics will need to have:

- a reception area which is easily accessible for patients and secure for staff;
- a waiting area with supplies of general information/leaflets;
- toilets;

- access to water and possibly tea and coffee for patients;
- adequate rooms for all personnel;
- notes storage and preparation area;
- a dedicated counselling room with all relevant literature available;
- store rooms;
- a phlebotomy area;
- resuscitation equipment;
- an ultrasound machine (ideally).

Ideally each room in a general clinic should have:

- a desk with an appropriately programmed PC;
- four chairs;
- adequate supplies of relevant paperwork that are checked daily;
- a curtained off area adjacent to, or with a couch, where the patients can change in privacy;
- a couch that is of variable height;
- a light source;
- adequate hand washing facilities (separate from the curtained area);
- clinical waste and normal waste bins;
- a bag/bin for instruments;
- gloves, sterile and non-sterile, in all sizes and a central store of latex free gloves;
- aprons;
- tissues;
- sanitary pads;
- a trolley/cupboard that contains:
  (a) lubricating jelly;
  (b) HVS and chlamydia swabs;
  (c) spatula, brushes, slides, transport boxes and fixatives for cervical smears;
  (d) speculums- Cusco's and Sims in varying sizes;
  (e) sponge holding forceps;
  (f) endometrial samplers;
  (g) IUCD packs that contain: uterine sound, dilators, and Tenaculum; sponge holding forceps; scissors; cotton wool; a galipot.
  (h) a selection of ring pessaries;
  (i) a selection of vaginal dilators;
  (j) betadine.

There should also be separate trolleys set up for specialist clinics such as uro-gynaecology and implants (see *Boxes 1.7* and *1.8*).

| Box 1.7 | Equipment for outpatients |
| --- | --- |

| General clinic requirements | Consulting rooms |
| --- | --- |
| Reception area | Desk with computer |
| Waiting area | Four chairs |
| Information/leaflets racks | Investigation request forms |
| Toilets (including disabled) | Prescription charts |
| Access to refreshments | Admission forms |
| Adequate rooms for all personnel | Curtained off patient change area |
| Notes storage and preparation area | Private examination area with basin |
| Computers and printers as required | |
| Counseling room with relevant literature | Variable height couch |
| Store rooms | Light source |
| Phlebotomy area | Clinical and normal waste bins |
| Resuscitation equipment | Bag/bin for instruments |
| CSSD room | All sizes of sterile and non-sterile gloves |
| Dirty utility | Aprons |

## One-stop clinics

With the introduction of new technologies, it is now possible to perform some procedures in the outpatients setting that would have previously been performed in the day surgery setting. It is therefore important when designing clinics to make some arrangement for the provision of one-stop clinics.

The development of one-stop clinics is associated with a decreased risk for women associated with a general anaesthetic, an increase in diagnostic accuracy, and a reduction in costs to the department, the patient and the patient's employer.

| Box 1.8 | Set up of clinic trolley |
| --- | --- |

| Contents of trolleys/cupboards | Additional contents for specialist clinics |
| --- | --- |
| Lubricating jelly | Lignocaine/oxypressin |
| HVS and chlamydia swabs | Syringes and needles (dental) |
| Spatula, brushes, fixative for Cx smear | Instilla gel and quills |
| Slides, pencil transport boxes | Gauze swabs and cotton wool balls |
| Cusco and Sims speculums | Endometrial samplers |
| Endometrial samplers | Silver nitrate sticks |
| Sponge holding forceps | IUCD packs: |
| | • tenaculum, uterine sound, dilators; |
| | • scissors, cotton wool, galipot; |
| | • selection of IUCD and IUS |
| Ring pessaries in various sizes | |
| Selection of vaginal dilators | Acetic acid/iodine |
| Betadine | Small and large curettes |
| | Small and large polyp forceps |
| | Wintertons' speculums. |

In a single appointment the patient can have a full history taken and an examination performed, followed by an ultrasound scan and/or a procedure as necessary. The appointment may last up to 2 hours but the patient will ideally leave with a diagnosis and a management plan or may have been fully treated and discharged.

There should be enough space in a one-stop clinic for:

- an ultrasound room;
- a consulting room;
- a procedure room.

These three rooms should ideally intercommunicate to allow the patient to move from one to the other without passing through a communal area. This allows one or more patients to be seen at the same time, with the ultrasonographer and the lead clinician seeing patients in parallel. It also allows for easy communication between professionals. The flow through the one-stop clinic is shown in *Figure 1. 3.*

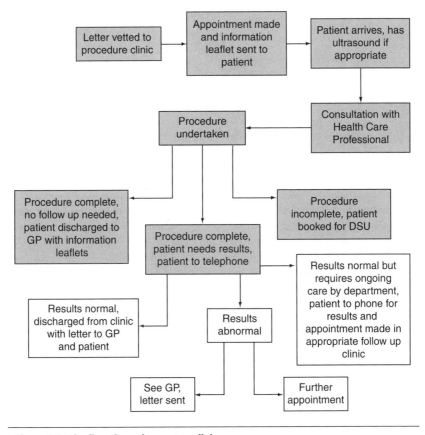

**Figure 1.3. The flow through one-stop clinic**

## Referral and clinic profile

The clinics should be able to accommodate a maximum of 12 patients each session, each with a 30 minute slot.

Patients who are suitable for the clinics are those whose referral letter suggests: cervical polyps or other abnormality: abnormal vaginal bleeding; post-coital bleeding; vulval problems (*Box 1.9*).

It is important that the referral letter is carefully vetted to plan the clinic case mix. It is not possible to perform 12 hysteroscopies in one clinic unless the department can afford four or more hysteroscopes and is allowed to decontaminate and sterilize the equipment in the clinic. The process for dealing with referral letters has been discussed at the beginning of this chapter and this is where patients who are suitable for a one-stop clinic can be identified.

| Box 1.9 | Conditions suitable for one-stop procedure clinic |
|---|---|

- Cervical polyps/ectropion
- Abnormal vaginal bleeding:
  IMB;
  PCB;
  Bleeding on HRT;
  Menorrhagia.
- Abnormal ultrasound scan:
  Endometrium >15 mm (premenopausal), >8 mm on HRT, >5 mm postmenopausal (consider rapid access clinic);
  Endometrial polyp/irregular uterine cavity.
- Vulval problems:
  Vulval dystrophy;
  Ulceration of vulva (Rapid Access Clinic);
  Bartholins abscess;
  Labial sebaceous cysts.

## Results management

A record should be kept in the clinic of all samples sent to histology and other investigations. A dedicated telephone line for the patients to ring for results and to discuss further management is very effective and efficient. The patients are asked to ring at a specific time 2 weeks after their appointment. Allowing patients access to specialist help at a dedicated time avoids the need, in some patients, for a repeated visit to outpatients and gives them support and help if problems arise.

The benefits of this service are that it saves time for the patients and the clinic staff. It is cost effective and allows for shorter follow-up lists of patients, which frees more clinic spaces for new patients (see *Boxes 1.10* and *1.11*).

| Box 1.10 | Results management from one-stop clinics |
|---|---|

- All one-stop clinics should have no patients returning for results
- If patients need appointments to review the treatment effectiveness then appointments should be made in the appropriate clinic
- Patients who have had investigations/tests taken should be advised to ring for results 2 weeks after the clinic appointment
- The patient should be given the results letter (*Box 1.11*)
- A record will be kept in the minor procedure room of all patients who will ring for results. This will be collected weekly
- Once the patient rings the results will be given
- If normal a letter will be sent to the patient and the GP and the original management plan adhered to
- If abnormal a further appointment may be made to discuss the results or they will be discussed with the consultant in charge and a letter sent to the GP and to the patient
- At the end of each help line the NP will review the results of the patients that have not rung and send letters to the GP and patient as appropriate

| Box 1.11 | Results letter |
|---|---|

Please reply to

Tel:

Fax:

Dear............................,

Patient sticker.

Following your visit today we have taken the following tests:

| Specimen | taken |
|---|---|
| FBC | |
| Oestrogen | |
| Prolactin | |
| LH/FSH | |
| Testosterone | |
| Endometrial biopsy | |
| Smear | |
| MSU | |
| Vulval biopsy | |
| Cervical biopsy | |
| Ultrasound | |
| Bone scan | |
| Other | |

In order to get your results and discuss any further clinic appointments please can you ring the results help line

**On _____ extension**

**On Date**

**Between time**

**Please note that results are not available at any other time**

## Staffing

Adequately trained staff must run the clinics. Ideally this should be a consultant doctor or nurse but may be a staff grade or associate specialist. It is wise to run the clinic alongside a consultant clinic in case additional medical help is required and/or advice is needed for future management. An appropriately trained nurse and /or health care assistant is needed to chaperone and assist. They should be trained in any maintenance, upkeep and sterilization procedures required. In addition they should be familiar with all the instruments and packs used in the clinic.

## Business planning

When setting up a clinic there needs to be a robust business plan to deal with the expensive outlay for equipment needed and future recurring costs (*Boxes 1.12* and *1.13*).

The following should be considered:

The benefits for the patients:

- single visit;
- no risk from a general anaesthetic;
- less disruption to work/ domestic arrangements.

Benefits for the hospital:

- reduction in the number of procedures in the day surgery unit;
- cost reduction.

Equipment needed:

- procedures couch;
- hysterscopes in varying sizes and if possible with operating channels and snares and scissors;
- a light source;
- carbon dioxide Hysterosufflator or normal saline;
- diathermy machine with patient pads, loops and balls;
- ultrasound machine;
- smoke extractor;
- colposcope;
- matt cuscoes with extractor channel;

| Box 1.12 The business case for one-stop clinics | |
|---|---|
| **Data required** | |
| Number of day cases | Diagnostic hysteroscopices |
| | Endometrial biopsies/D&Cs |
| | Vulval biopsies |
| | Cervical polypectomies |
| | Cervical cauterization |
| **Number thought to be suitable for one-stop clinic** | |
| Costings | Day case surgery including staff time |
| | Capital costs of equipment |
| | Recurrent costs for staffing |
| Advantages to patients | Single visit |
| | No risk from a general anaesthetic |
| | Immediate discussion of findings |
| | Fully awake and alert |
| | Less disruption to work/domestic arrangements |
| Advantages for PCT/ Hospital Trust | Reduced costs |
| | Reduced waiting list for day surgery |

| Box 1.13 | Equipment needed for Minor Procedures clinic |

**Ultrasound room**
Procedures couch
Desk and three chairs
Ultrasound machines (with Doppler)
Thermal imager linked to ultrasound machine
PC and printer to enter ultrasound report
Condoms for vaginal probe
Alcohol wipes for probe
Gloves

**Minor Procedures room**

Hysterscopes in varying sizes and if possible with operating
channels Hysteroscopic snares and scissors
A light source
Carbon dioxide Hysterosufflator or normal saline
Diathermy machine with patient pads
Diathermy loops and balls
Cryocautery machine
Smoke extractor
Colposcope
Matt cuscoes with extractor channel
TV monitor
Video printer
Camera
Decontamination and sterilization of instruments
Trolley as per special clinics (*Box 1.8*)

- TV monitor;
- video printer;
- camera;
- instrument decontamination and sterilization equipment.

It is, however, becoming increasingly difficult to undertake local decontamination within clinical areas and this will need to be established and agreed by the Trust. If it is not possible to undertake this locally then there are cost implications as the number of instruments required is increased in line with the CSSD turnaround time.

The video printer is important for accurate record keeping and clinical governance. It is also important to provide for training of the staff prior to starting the clinic and on-going professional development

Alongside the equipment and in addition to the normal clinic trolleys there should be a trolley that contains the following:

- Lignocaine or oxypressin;
- syringes and needles or dental syringes and needles;
- instilla gel and quills;

- gauze swabs and cotton wool balls;
- Os finders;
- IUCD removal hooks;
- selection of IUCD and IUS;
- endometrial samplers;
- silver nitrate sticks;
- sutures and suturing packs;
- blades and handles;
- Betadine;
- acetic acid;
- small and large curettes;
- small and large polyp forceps;
- punch biopsy forceps;
- cervical dilators;
- uterine sounds;
- sponge holders;
- Winterton's speculums.

The following recurrent costs need to be considered:

- nursing staff;
- ultrasonographer;
- maintenance contracts;
- repair and replacement costs.

The negotiation over costing the clinic should include the cost saving from the day surgery unit. The number of cases can be accurately predicted from the number of diagnostic hysteroscopies performed in the day surgery unit plus a case-mix review of the referral letters and cases seen in clinics.

## The role of the rapid access clinic

The rapid access clinic is similar to the one-stop clinic in set up, design and equipment needed. The difference is that patients who are referred as urgent or query cancer will be referred directly into this clinic, which should be run by a gynaecological oncologist. Not all patients will need to have a procedure in this clinic, but the majority of patients will require an ultrasound prior to being seen in the clinic. In line with Government targets most hospitals will now have in place a system for dealing with urgent patients who meet the 2-week wait criteria. This is no different in gynaecology and the urgent patients are normally referred with:

- post-menopausal bleeding (PMB);
- ovarian cysts;
- vulval problems;
- invasive cervical cancer on smear.

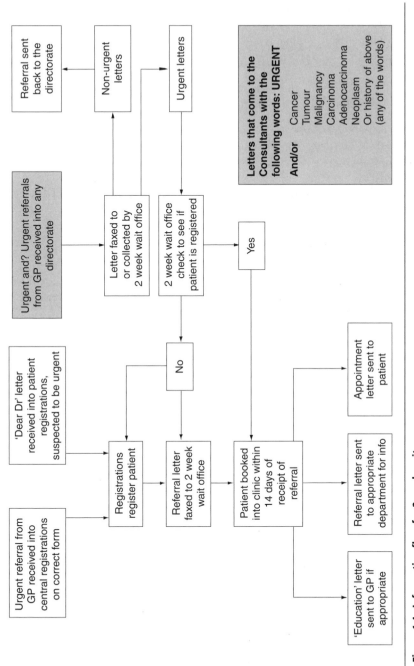

**Letters that come to the Consultants with the following words: URGENT**

**And/or** Cancer
Tumour
Malignancy
Carcinoma
Adenocarcinoma
Neoplasm
Or history of above
(any of the words)

Referral sent back to the directorate

Non-urgent letters

Urgent letters

Urgent and? Urgent referrals from GP received into any directorate

Letter faxed to or collected by 2 week wait office

2 week wait office check to see if patient is registered

Yes

No

'Dear Dr' letter received into patient registrations, suspected to be urgent

Registrations register patient

Referral letter faxed to 2 week wait office

Patient booked into clinic within 14 days of receipt of referral

Appointment letter sent to patient

Urgent referral from GP received into central registrations on correct form

Referral letter sent to appropriate department for info

'Education' letter sent to GP if appropriate

**Figure 1.4. Information flow for 2 week wait**

*Figure 1.4* shows how the process for these referral letters varies from that detailed at the start of this chapter.

To ensure that the clinic is efficient most patients will need investigations or tests prior to their appointment. These are normally sent out with the clinic letters.

If the referral is for an ovarian cyst or pelvic mass then the following should have been performed prior to the appointment:

- ultrasound scan (USS);
- CA 125;
- CEA;
- CA199;
- occasionally it may be necessary to also perform- AFP, Beta HCG, LDH (see Chapter 2).

For PMB:

- USS.

The rapid access clinic will be seeing new and follow-up patients but should not see patients who have known benign disease, these patients should be referred, if necessary, back to their GP or to other general gynaecologists.

# Clinical Gynaecological Management of Outpatients

# 2 | Menstrual Dysfunction

## Menorrhagia

### Introduction

Menorrhagia is a very common complaint and accounts for 50% of all referrals to a specialist. Five percent of women aged 30–49 consult their GP each year with menorrhagia. Recent guidelines from the RCOG have supplied a format for investigation and treatment of this condition within primary care prior to referral to secondary health care services.

This chapter will look at the interface between primary and secondary care and how they can work together to maximize the effectiveness and efficiency for looking after women who complain of menorrhagia.

### Definition

Menorrhagia is defined as a complaint of heavy cyclical menstrual bleeding over several consecutive cycles in a woman of reproductive years (age 25–49).

### Referral from primary care

The introduction of the RCOG guidelines allows many women with menorrhagia to be treated in the community. The responsibility of the gynaecology service lies in ensuring that women referred to the secondary services have been adequately investigated and treated prior to referral. A proforma (see *Figure 2.1*) has been shown to be a useful tool both for primary and secondary care. The proforma is completed by the GP and sent to the outpatient department. A nurse practitioner checks that all parts of the proforma have been completed and that the patient has been fully investigated and/or treated appropriately within primary care.

An appointment for the minor procedures clinic should then be sent particularly for women aged over 40 or where the ultrasound scan shows an abnormality of the endometrium. If the woman has been referred by the Community Gynaecology Service then she may have already had an endometrial biopsy in which case it is important to obtain a copy of the histology report. An information leaflet is sent to all women (*Figure 2.2*).

Women who have a normal ultrasound scan but have failed all medical treatment on the proforma can be sent an appointment for the general gynaecology outpatients (See *Box 2.1*).

| Name of patient | DOB | GPs stamp (Name/address/code) |

Name of patient                    DOB

Address



NHS Number

Hospital Number

GPs stamp (Name/address/code)

---

**History**

Cycle: Days of bleeding/cycle length (dl–dl) ....../......    Clots ☐    Flooding ☐

**Regular/Irregular**          **Dysmenorrhoea Yes/No**              **Dyspareunia Yes/No**

**IUCD *in situ*  Type**                              **Interested in future fertility Yes/No**

Smear        Date        Result              Uterine size <10/52 ☐  >10/52 ☐

Hb           Date        Result              Cervical polyp Yes/No

Other medication:                    Relevant PMH

---

**Treatment:**   Mefenemic acid            Yes/No        Duration

Tranexemic acid           Yes/No        Duration

Combined ocp              Yes/No        Duration

Mirena IUS                Yes/No        Duration

Long-acting progestogens  Yes/No        Duration

Further investigations prior to referral:

---

Transvaginal ultrasound scan:

Endometrium      thickness:                    Appearance: Normal/abnormal

Myometrium:      Normal/heterogeneous/fibroids

Ovaries:         Normal/Polycystic ovaries/Ovarian cyst > 4cm

---

**Figure 2.1.  Proforma for referral of women aged 25-49 complaining of heavy cyclical bleeding (Menorrhagia)**

**Women's health services**

## MINOR PROCEDURE CLINIC

You have been invited to attend the minor procedure clinic, this leaflet is to explain the function of the clinic and what will happen to you during your visit.

## AIM OF THE CLINIC

This is a one-stop clinic for consultation, diagnosis and treatment within one clinic.

This clinic is a gynaecology outpatient clinic where you will see a Health Care professional who will carry out the necessary investigations, explain what is wrong and offer you advice or treatment. The clinic sees women who have problems with the following:

Abnormal vaginal bleeding – heavy periods
- irregular periods
- bleeding between periods
- bleeding after intercourse
- bleeding after the menopause.

Cervical polyps
Heavy/offensive vaginal discharge
Cysts or other problems with the vagina/ vulva.

## WHAT INVESTIGATIONS MAY BE CARRIED OUT:

### Abnormal vaginal bleeding

- You may have an ultrasound scan, vaginally.
- Physical examination.
- Hysteroscopy under local anesthetic.
- Biopsy of the lining of the womb.

### Cervical polyps
- Ultrasound scan
- Physical examination
- Removal of the polyp.

### Heavy discharge
- Examination.
- Swabs taken from the cervix.
- Heating of the cells of the cervix under local anaesthetic.

### Cysts or vaginal/vulva problems.
- Removal under local anaesthetic.

The type of investigations that are carried out in the clinic are listed below:

- An ultrasound involves having a small probe inserted into the vagina to produce a picture of your womb and ovaries, this does not hurt.

**Figure 2.2.** *continued overleaf*

- A speculum examination involves the same instrument as when you have a smear test and some swabs may be taken at this time.
- A hysteroscopy involves the passing a telescope-like instrument through the neck of your womb to look at the inside of the womb. To do this it may be necessary to give you an injection of local anaesthetic in to the cervix, which may sting.
- Biopsies can also be taken from the neck of the womb, the cervix, and from the lining of the womb. These will then be sent off to the laboratory to be examined.

If you do not wish to have the procedures in outpatients we will admit you to the day surgery unit.

### Will I have pain?

Some of the procedures may require the use of local anaesthetic. This does not mean that you will be put to sleep so you can eat and drink normally before your appointment. After some procedures you may have some pain afterwards. We would suggest that you took some normal painkillers about an hour before your appointment.

### Will I have bleeding?

Some procedures can cause bleeding from the injection sites or biopsy sites. This is not heavy and will last a few days. It is important not to use tampons for this bleed.

### GOING HOME

As some of the procedures involve the use of local anaesthetic, we would advise that you arrange for some one to take you home and take the rest of the day off work.

The average time you will spend in clinic is about 2 hours depending on which procedure you had performed.

**If you are bleeding please contact the nurse on the number below as it can affect certain procedures.**

All biopsies taken are sent to the laboratories to be checked under the microscope. We will either make you a follow-up appointment, or you can telephone our result line or we will write to you and your GP with the result.

**If you have enquires then please contact**

**If you need to change or cancel the appointment the please contact the outpatients supervisor on**

Figure 2.2. Women's health services

| Box 2.1 | Ultrasound findings in menorrhagia |
|---|---|
| **Normal ultrasound (D5–D8)** | **Abnormal ultrasound (D5–D8)** |
| Endometrium <12 mm | Endometrium >12 mm |
| Regular endometrial outline | Irregular endometrial outline, cystic spaces, ? polyp, submucosal fibroid |
| Normal uterine size | Increased uterine size |
| Normal myometrium | Heterogeneous myometrium, fibroid change, fibroids |
| No adnexal masses | Presence of an ovarian cyst |

## Consultation and investigation

As in all consultations it is important to check the patients history and confirm that the problem of heavy bleeding has persisted. If the haemoglobin (Hb) is normal it is essential to make some subjective measures of menstrual loss including a history of duration of bleeding, number of days that are perceived to be heavy, the type of protection used and how often it is changed. Confirm that the cycle is still regular and that there is no intermenstrual or post-coital bleeding (see Oncology chapter). Further details about dysmenorrhoea and dyspareunia should be taken. A complete past medical history and medical history can be of help since women with a past history of thrombophilia who are on long-term anticoagulant therapy may have menorrhagia with no other underlying pathology.

If the ultrasound is normal and the patient is not anaemic check that she has had a recent smear and do a full vaginal and abdominal examination. If she is over the age of 40 then she should have an endometrial biopsy.

Objective measures include pictorial blood assessment charts. The patient may be reassured to know that her menstrual loss is not excessive and that there is no underlying pathology.

If the ultrasound is abnormal or the woman is anaemic (Hb <11) the patient should have a hysteroscopy under local anesthesia and an endometrial biopsy. If a submucosal fibroid or endometrial polyp (*Figure 2.3*) is found then the patient should be placed on the waiting list for day surgery. If the endometrial polyp is less than 1cm in size then it can be safely removed in outpatients using a small (3 mm) operating hysteroscope or with polyp forceps. Women with a submucosal fibroid should be given LHRH analogues for at least 6 weeks prior to the procedure.

Following the procedure the patient should be followed up at 3 months and advised according to her continuing symptoms.

If the hysteroscopy and endometrial biopsy are normal then secondary medical treatment, continuous progestogens (Medroxy progesterone acetate, Norethisterone, Gestrinone), Mirena IUS, Danazol, LHRH analogues with non-bleed add back HRT for 6 months should be given (*Box 2.2*). If these do not achieve a satisfactory outcome then the patient can be offered surgery,

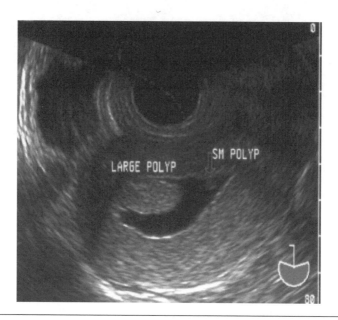

**Figure 2.3. Saline transvaginal ultrasound scan of endometrial polyp**

endometrial ablation or hysterectomy (see *Figure 2.4*). The commonest reason for failure of treatment is underlying adenomyosis, which commonly coexists with endometriosis and fibroids. Most of these patients fail all forms of treatment with constant break through bleeding.

# Benign causes of intermenstrual bleeding and post-coital bleeding

## Introduction

Intermenstrual bleeding (IMB) and post-coital bleeding (PCB) are common in women and can occur regularly or intermittently. In premenopausal women they rarely signify major pathology although both can be associated with the possibility of underlying malignancy. It is therefore important that all women with these symptoms have malignancy ruled out as a cause before considering benign conditions.

The investigation and management of these symptoms can be undertaken in a one-stop clinic.

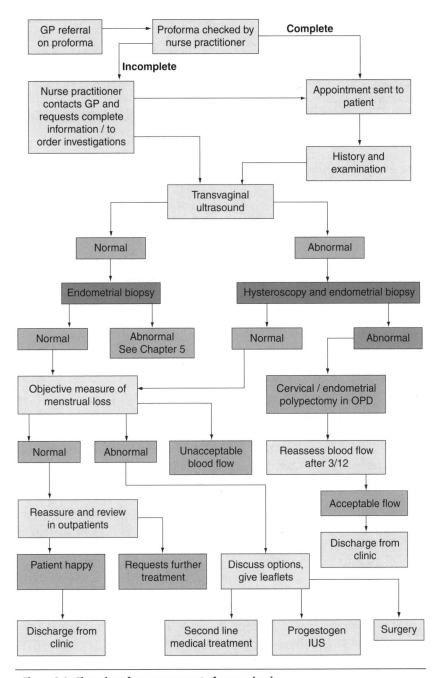

**Figure 2.4. Flow chart for management of menorrhagia**

| Box 2.2 | Medical treatment | |
|---|---|---|
| **Continuous high dose progestogens** | | |
| Medroxyprogesterone | 10 mg tds | |
| Norethisterone | 5 mg tds | |
| Gestrinone | 10 mg b.d | |
| Danazol | 200 mg b.d | |
| **LHRH analogues** | | |
| Goserelin | 3.5 mg mthly | |
| **Add back therapy** | | |
| Tibolone | 1/day | |
| **Mirena IUS** | | |
| | Single insertion lasts 3–5 years | |

## Definitions

- IMB is defined as any bleeding that occurs within a regular menstrual cycle but not at menstruation.
- PCB is defined as bleeding after sexual intercourse.

## Evaluation

It is vital to fully evaluate women who present with these symptoms since a minority will have a malignancy. The evaluation should include history and investigations

- Complete history – gynaecological, obstetric, medical and surgical.
- A complete menstrual and contraceptive history.
- The duration of the problem including amount of bleeding, type of bleeding and when this occurs.
- A pelvic examination.
- Cervical smear.
- A full GU screen if indicated.
- A vaginal ultrasound.

With appropriate management in general practice gynaecology referrals should be limited to women who have repeated episodes of IMB or PCB.

Once these patients have been referred to the outpatients department they should ideally be seen within the one-stop diagnostic and treatment clinics. The clinic should have the facility to undertake ultrasound, hysteroscopy, and colposcopy.

A full gynaecological and obstetric history should be taken focussing on the menstrual history, contraceptive history and sexual history in particular. Examination must include a pelvic examination, examination of the cervix with a smear test and swabs from the vagina and cervix including chlamydia.

The patients should have a transvaginal ultrasound and an endometrial biopsy (under 40). A hysteroscopy should be performed if the scan is abnormal or if the woman is over 40 to determine if the endometrium is normal. The main role of these outpatient procedures is diagnostic but with the increase in technology there is an increasing role for treatment procedures such as endometrial polypectomy.

## Common causes of IMB and PCB

The common causes of IMB and PCB are listed in *Box 2.3*

- **Physiological causes.** The physiological causes are related to the normal fluctuations of oestrogen and progesterone in the menstrual cycle. A large rise in oestrogen in the follicular phase followed by a fall immediately post-ovulation can give rise to the endometrium losing its hormonal support. This can lead to consistent mid-cycle IMB.
- **Cervical ectropion.** The cervix is composed of two types of epithelium. One of these the columnar epithelium is usually inside the cervical canal, while the squamous epithelium is over the outer part of the cervix and is visible. These two epithelium meet at the squamo-columnar junction (S-CJ), which moves into and out of the cervical canal in response to hormonal changes. An ectropion occurs when this S-CJ moves on to the surface of the cervix. The columnar epithelium that becomes visible looks like a reddened, inflamed area. This epithelium is fragile and can bleed easily on contact especially after intercourse. There is no need to treat this if the smear is normal unless the woman considers the symptoms to be a problem. This is a common finding in women on the combined oral contraceptive pill (COCP). An ectropion can be the cause of a persistent vaginal discharge that may be blood stained if there is cervicitis present as well. If the symptoms are problematic the use of cryocautery or diathermy is recommended.

| Box 2.3 | Common causes of IMB and PCB |
|---|---|

- Physiological
- Cervical ectropion
- Oral contraceptives
- Vulvitis
- Recent insertion of an IUS
- Progestrogen only pill
- Depo provera
- Cervical polyp
- Submucosal fibroid
- Endometrial hyperplasia
- Endometritis/PID
- Concurrent medical conditions

- **Oral contraceptives.** Some women do not absorb the COCP well. This leads to reports of IMB. This is common with the first few packets of starting the pill and should resolve spontaneously. If it does not then a different pill should be prescribed.
- **Progesteron only pill (POP).** Women on the POP also report IMB. It is important to check that she is taking the pill correctly. If the problem persists then changing to a different progesterone only pill may help resolve the problem.
- **Cervical polyps/fibroids.** Cervical polyps may give rise to both IMB and PCB. The treatment is to remove the polyp and to check if there are any further endometrial polyps, which may compound the problem. The treatment for fibroids is normally to resect them as a day case.
- **Vulvitis.** This can be treated with a prescription of antifungal medication.

- **Endometrial hyperplasia.** If there is a diagnosis of endometrial hyperplasia then this needs to be treated with progestogen.
- **Endometritis/PID.** Intrauterine infections secondary to sexually transmitted diseases including gonorrhoea and chlamydia or following an evacuation of retained products of conception can lead to IMB and PCB if cervicitis is present.
- **Concurrent medical conditions.** These can play a part in these conditions. Women who are epileptic or who have been on antibiotics whilst taking the COCP commonly get IMB or breakthrough bleeding and need a higher dose pill and/or additional contraception until the symptom has stopped. Women on warfarin or long-term anticoagulants are also more prone to IMB.

# Fibroids

## Management of fibroids

Fibroids are benign leiomyomas arising in the uterus. They are relatively common, particularly in women of Afro-Caribbean origin. They vary in size and site and therefore in their presentation. They can be multiple or single and the uterus may grow very large indeed (*Figure 2.5*). The side effects of treatment are

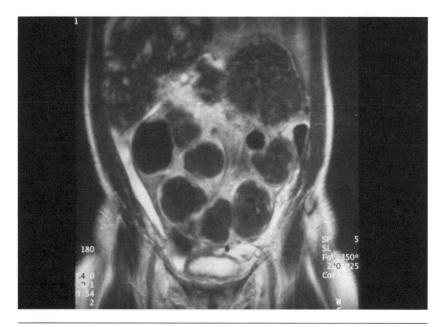

**Figure 2.5. MRI of multiple intramural and subserosal fibroids**

profound and must be weighed up very carefully before embarking on invasive methods of treatment.

The symptoms associated with fibroids vary according to their size and site. They do have a natural life cycle that is affected by the age of the woman and pregnancy.

## Sites of fibroids

- Surface of the uterus – Subserosal
- In the myometrium – Intramural (*Figure 2.5*)
- Indenting the endometrium – Submucosal (*Figure 2.6*)
- In the endometrial cavity – Fibroid polyp (*Figure 2.7*)

For symptoms associated with fibroids see *Box 2.4*. Some women have no symptoms from their fibroids even when they are very large. The risk of fibroids becoming malignant is less than one in a thousand. Intervention in these women should bear in mind the relative risks and the cultural needs of the women.

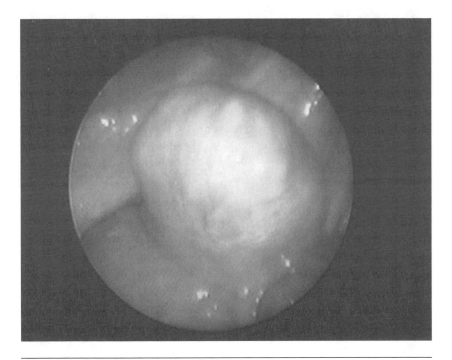

**Figure 2.6. Submucosal fibroid**

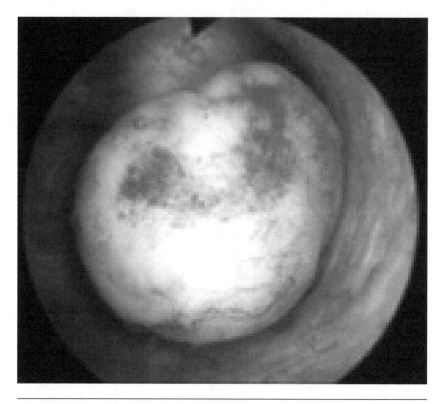

**Figure 2.7. Hysteroscopic image of a fibroid polyp**

| Box 2.4 | Symptoms associated with fibroids |
|---|---|
| • Menorrhagia | |
| • Dysmenorrhoea | |
| • Abdominal pain | |
| • Pressure symptoms (bladder/rectum) | |
| • Subfertility | |
| • Miscarriage | |
| • Premature labour | |

## Subserosal fibroids

- **Abdominal pain.** if they are undergoing degeneration. This can cause severe pain requiring admission for adequate pain relief. The duration of the pain varies according to the size of the fibroid, its site and the individual. The majority will settle down after a few days although there may be recurrent bouts until the process of degeneration is complete. This tends to affect women as they approach the menopause or during pregnancy.
- **Pressure symptoms.** The symptoms depend on the site of the fibroid. Posterior wall fibroids, which are near the isthmus or cervix may cause

pressure on the rectum leading to tenesmus or constipation. Anterior wall fibroids can put pressure on the bladder leading to frequency, nocturia and incomplete emptying which may increase the risk of urinary tract infections.

## Intramural fibroids

- **Menorrhagia.** Blood flow may be greater in the presence of fibroids because of the inability of the vessels supplying the endometrium overlying the intramural fibroid to undergo the usual progestogenic changes.
- **Dysmenorrhoea.** The myometrium may contract during menstruation in order to try and push the intramural fibroid into the cavity so it can be expelled. Dysmenorrhoea is more commonly associated with adenomyosis which often coexists with fibroids causing generalized enlargement of the uterus with multiple small fibroids and heterogeneous change (*Figure 2.8*) on ultrasound scan or MRI.

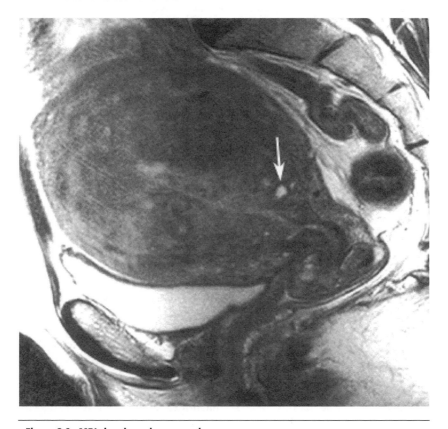

**Figure 2.8. MRI showing adenomysosis**

- **Subfertility.** Intramural fibroids have been shown to be associated with subfertility presumably because they interfere with implantation or partially or completely block the fallopian tubes.
- **Miscarriage.** Early miscarriage may be secondary to problems with implantation, second trimester miscarriages and/or premature labour may arise secondary to degeneration which causes myometrial contractions.

## Submucosal fibroids and fibroid polyps

- **Dysmenorrhoea.** This type of fibroid is most commonly associated with dysmenorrhoea as the uterus tries to expel the fibroid through the cervix, which it commonly succeeds in doing.
- **Menorrhagia.** These fibroids are by definition covered by endometrium. A sphere increases the surface area of endometrium four-fold. This increase in surface area together with a vascular bed that does not respond normally to the effects of progesterone leads to very heavy prolonged bleeding. These women often present with severe anaemia.

## Investigations

- Abdominal and pelvic examination
- Ultrasound scan and or MRI
- Full blood count

## Treatment

The treatment of fibroids depends on the symptoms. Asymptomatic women can be safely left untreated with annual checks on the size of the uterus to try and detect sarcomatous change, which is very rare.

Women who are symptomatic need to be advised very carefully about their options (Figure 2.9).

Medical treatment with LHRH analogues is effective in shrinking the size of fibroids. However, the side effects of hot flushes, reduced ability to concentrate and other menopausal symptoms can be significant. Pain is also quite common as the fibroid degenerates. The most important long-term side effect is loss of bone mass increasing the risk of fracture. Used for a short time the bone mass will be replaced but long-term (greater than 6 months) the remineralization of the bone may be impaired. Studies using non-oestrogenic add back therapy have shown that bone mass can be maintained and the menopausal symptoms minimized. Unfortunately within 6 months of ceasing treatment there is a return to significant symptomatology in the majority of women.

Important considerations for the woman include the inability to conceive whilst on treatment and the high probability that their symptoms will return when they stop treatment.

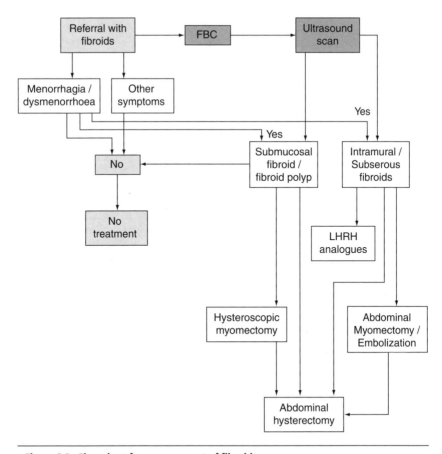

**Figure 2.9. Flow chart for management of fibroids**

LHRH analogues are very useful prior to surgery. They are essential for 3 months prior to undertaking a transcervical resection of a submucous fibroid or a fibroid polyp. Firstly the treatment reduces the size and vascularity of the fibroid thus reducing the risk of excess absorption of glycine making the procedure safer. LHRH also reduces the size of intramural and subserosal fibroids which may convert a midline scar for myomectomy or hysterectomy to a low transverse abdominal wound.

## Uterine artery embolization/laser ablation of fibroids

These procedures are relatively non-invasive and can be performed safely under local anaesthesia in the X-ray department. They are only undertaken in tertiary referral centres and are not without risks. Women with large multiple fibroids are at four-fold risk of requiring a hysterectomy following embolization compared with surgical myomectomy in experienced hands. The fibroids degenerate very rapidly causing intense pain which requires hospitalization. It is not known what the outcome of pregnancy is following the procedure but successful pregnancy has been reported in several series. Laser ablation is less well established and is still undergoing evaluation in research studies. Currently neither treatment is recommended in women who wish to preserve their fertility.

Surgical treatment involves myomectomy. Transcervical myomectomy is a highly successful procedure with low risks if preceded by 3 months of treatment with LHRH analogue. The treatment improves symptomatic menorrhagia and dysmenorrhoea and increases the chances of successful pregnancy.

Transabdominal myomectomy carries a small risk of hysterectomy (around 1%) but this largely depends on the number and site of the fibroids. A single fundal fibroid carries very little risk regardless of size, whilst multiple intramural fibroids particularly those involving the broad ligament and/or cervix carry a much higher risk. Women over the age of 42 might be better served with a hysterectomy but for strong cultural reasons women of Afro-Caribbean origin are very reluctant to have their uteruses removed and their wishes should be respected. The operation will relieve pressure symptoms and menorrhagia to the same extent in a 45-year-old woman as it will a 35-year-old woman. Therefore, the older woman should be offered a myomectomy as a valid alternative to hysterectomy.

# 3 Pelvic Pain and Dyspareunia

## Differential diagnosis of pelvic pain and dyspareunia

Pelvic pain is one of the commonest conditions referred to the gynaecology outpatients clinic. It can have a large number of underlying causes, some of which are easy to diagnose and treat. However, a large number of patients may end up without a physical/clinical name for their pain. Patients find this very frustrating and often think gynaecologists are trying to infer that their pain is imaginary or that they are psychologically disturbed.

It is important that the clinician seeing the patient is sympathetic and believes the patient as she tells her story. The initial rapport with the patient will determine whether or not she will accept the explanation for her pain if no physical cause is found. It is important that a full psychosexual history is taken in the first or second consultation, however, this will only be possible if the patient trusts the clinician. Nursing staff can often be the member of the team to whom the patient confides their problems and it is therefore vital that the team members communicate with each other during and/or immediately after the consultation. If significant psychological or sexual problems are identified during the history taking then a referral to a psychologist or gynaecologist with a particular interest and training in psychosexual problems is recommended. Ideally a psychologist should form part of the team in gynaecology outpatients. Unfortunately it is often difficult to get this funded within the NHS, however, it can be argued for as part of a Mental Health Service for women which encompasses maternity, obstetrics and gynaecology.

Women with pelvic pain do not necessarily have a gynaecological cause for their pain and so the evaluation of the patient should include evaluation of other relevant systems.

## Evaluation of pelvic pain

### History

The history taking should start with a standard gynaecological history as well as details about the pain that include:

- Characteristics: site, time, duration and nature, particularly in relation to the menstrual cycle, how severe the pain is on an analogue score.
- Radiation of the pain.
- Associated relieving and aggravating factors.

- Past medical and surgical history, particularly pelvic surgery, previous sexually transmitted diseases or pelvic inflammatory disease, urinary tract problems.
- Past obstetric history including ectopic pregnancies and Caesarean sections.
- Social history should include an enquiry into the state of the patient's current relationships if she has one, whether her partner is supportive, is there a history of abuse or domestic violence within this or any previous relationships.
- System history should include bowel habit and relation to pain, urinary symptoms and bony problems.

### Dyspareunia

Pain on intercourse may be deep or superficial and it is important to establish the difference with the patient and get a clear and thorough history of the problem. The pain may vary depending on the position adopted during intercourse and advice on different positions can often be helpful. The length of time this has been a problem, the impact it may be having on the current relationship and past history of relationships, including possible abuse, are all important factors to explore and establish.

## Examination

The patient should have a full examination and a pelvic examination which should include the taking of a high vaginal swab and two cervical swabs to detect any infection including chlamydia. A note should also be taken of any vaginismus if the patient also complains of dyspareunia.

## Investigations

A transvaginal ultrasound is essential for all women presenting with pelvic pain. Any positive finding such as ovarian cysts should be treated accordingly and will not be dealt with in great detail in this chapter since the main diagnoses are dealt with in separate chapters. Other investigations such as MSU, colonoscopy or barium enema should be tailored to the individual history.

## Differential diagnosis

The particular features of the history, examination and investigations can be used to make a differential diagnosis for dyspareunia and pelvic pain. These are set out in *Table 3.1*.

If on system review there are significant urinary, bowel or skeletal symptoms then the patient should be referred to the appropriate specialist after arranging appropriate investigations (*Table 3.2*).

**Table 3.1.** Evaluation of pelvic pain and dyspareunia

| Diagnosis | History | Examination | Investigation | Treatment |
|---|---|---|---|---|
| **Genital tract** | | | | |
| Vaginismus | Superficial dyspareunia, history of abuse/rape is common | Unable to perform | None initially | Psychosexual counselling and/or vaginal dilators |
| Vulvodynia | Superficial dyspareunia, constant pain, feels like red-hot needles | Tender on two specific points at introitus. Rest NAD | None | Steroid cream, counselling |
| Vulval dystrophy | Vulval itching with or without bleeding | White plaques | Biopsy | Steroid cream |
| Prolapse | Dragging sensation with or without urinary GI symptoms | Cystocoele/rectocoele | Consider urodynamics | Surgery |
| **Uterus** | | | | |
| Fibroids – subserosal/intramural | Intermittent, constant pain, with or without menorrhagia, pressure symptoms | Enlarged irregular tender uterus | Site of fibroids on USS | Surgery/embolization/none |
| Submucosal | Dysmenorrhoea, intermittent, constant pain, with or without menorrhagia | Enlarged uterus, fibroid polyp in cervical canal | Present on USS | LHRH analogue + hysteroscopic resection of fibroid |
| Adenomyosis | Constant and crampy pain with period, menorrhagia, prolonged bleeding, resistant to medical treatment | Uniformly enlarged uterus, no discrete masses | Heterogenous fibroid change, multiple small fibroids | Medical treatment initially hysterectomy |
| **Fallopian tubes** | | | | |
| Chronic PID/Hydrosalpinx | Vaginal discharge, past history of PID | May be palpable but rare | Tubular structure on USS or normal. | Laparoscopy, adhesiolysis, salpingectomy |
| **Ovary** | | | | |
| Mittleschmerz pain | Midcycle pain, may have IMB, varies from cycle to cycle | Normal | Normal | Reassurance and/or laparoscopy to confirm |
| Ovarian cyst | Dull unilateral pain, may have exacerbations, may cause dyspareunia which varies with position, may be cyclical | >5 cm cyst may be palpable | Cyst seen on scan, may be able to identify its nature (haemorrhagic/simple/dermoid ovarian markers | Laparoscopy drainage and or removal of cyst. |
| **Peritoneum** | | | | |
| Endometriosis | Cyclical pain with menses, may have metastatic sites | Tender nodular uterosacral ligaments, ovarian endometriomas | USS often negative | Laparoscopy and diathermy followed by medical treatment. |
| Chronic pelvic pain | No relationship to cycle, often point to specific point of abdomen, variable aggravating and relieving factors, anorgasmic, post-coital ache | May be tender on vaginal examination | USS negative, may remark on dilated pelvic veins | Laparoscopy, 6 months high dose provera and counselling. |

**Table 3.2.** Evaluation of other systems

| Diagnosis | History | Examination | Investigation | Treatment |
|---|---|---|---|---|
| **GI system** | | | | |
| Irritable bowel syndrome | Variable bowel motion, pain relieved when bowels open, usually left sided pain, related to diet, no relationship with menstrual cycle | NAD in all systems | Colonoscopy – NAD Laparoscopy – NAD | High fibre diet Exclude dietary factors one by one to see which makes things worse Colpermin Lactulose/Fybogel |
| Diverticulitis | Constipation, intermittent pain | NAD | Colonoscopy – diverticuli seen Laparoscopy – NAD | As above Refer to gastroenterologist |
| Herniae | Pain worse on standing, coughing. May notice a lump no gynaecological symptoms | Inguinal hernia present. Check carefully for femoral hernia | All NAD | Refer to general surgeon |
| **Urinary tract** | | | | |
| Chronic cystitis | Recurrent UTIs Pain made worse on micturition, associated loin pain, central suprapubic ache | NAD usually | MSU positive Cystoscopy Laparoscopy – NAD | Depends on results of investigations. Refer to urogynaecologist or urologist |
| Urinary reflux | Pain worse on micturition, radiates to loin | Tender in loin sometimes | MSU –ve Micturating IVU – +ve | Refer urologist |
| Renal stone | Intermittent severe pain, radiating from loin to pelvis | Loin tenderness | Stone visible on IVU or plain abdominal X-ray or USS | Refer to urologist for lithotripsy |
| **Skeletal system** | | | | |
| Slipped vertebral disc | Pain worse on walking, sciatica, history of chronic back pain | Tender over disc space, reduced straight leg raising | Lumbar spine X-ray may be positive | Refer to orthopaedic surgeon |

## Treatment

The treatment of pelvic pain and dyspareunia will depend on the underlying cause. The majority of those mentioned in *Tables 3.1* and *3.2* are explored in other chapters.

For treatment of vaginismus in the outpatient clinic the main facility required is a nurse practitioner or doctor skilled in teaching the use of vaginal dilators.

The patient must be in a private room and feel secure that no-one will suddenly walk in. The following should then be undertaken:

- The dilators should be sterile when first used but can then be cleaned in soapy water, rinsed and dried.

- The smallest dilator should be tried first since failure with the first attempt can mean that the patient will never use them.
- The nurse should show the patient how to lubricate the dilator with jelly
- The nurse should then explain the natural course that the vagina takes towards the small of the patients back so that the dilator can slide in more easily.
- The dilator should be held at its open end between thumb and middle finger and the tip gently placed at the introitus. Ideally the patient should do this herself but sometimes the nurse or doctor needs to start the process to give confidence that this is not embarrassing or painful.
- The patient should now be encouraged to hold the dilator herself and gradually insert it in to her vagina. She should stop as soon as it becomes painful.
- If the patient stops then the nurse can ask her to describe the pain and/or the reasons she has stopped. Further encouragement should be given to try and insert the dilator a little further.
- If this is not possible then the patient should be asked to take the dilator out and put it back in again a few times until she feels more comfortable. She can be left alone to continue the exercises.
- Once she is comfortable with the process then she should be given that dilator and the one size bigger and told to return in 2-3 weeks time able to use the larger dilator but not to worry if she can't as everyone takes a different length of time to do this.
- If appropriate she should be referred to a psychosexual counsellor.
- On the follow-up visit a review of how far the patient has got is undertaken. A frank discussion about any difficulties she may be having and their cause should be held before giving her the next two sizes of dilator.
- Generally the patient makes faster progress with the larger dilators having overcome most of her fears and anxieties with the smaller ones.

For other treatments see *Table 3.1*.

# Management of endometriosis

## Introduction

Endometriosis is one of the most common conditions seen within the gynae-cology outpatients setting. It is difficult to know exactly how many women have endometriosis, as some women are asymptomatic. It is estimated that 3–7% of women age 20–45 have the disease. It is most common in this age group but can occur from ages 10 to 60.

## Definition

It is defined as the presence of tissue histologically similar to endometrium outside the uterine cavity and the myometrium, which responds to ovarian hormones in the same way as endometrium.

The definitive diagnosis for endometriosis is at laparoscopy when it is further classified into minimal, mild, moderate and severe. This classification is based on anatomical findings within the pelvis and bears little or no relation to the degree of suffering a woman may experience or to the effect it may have on her future fertility. The sites in which it may occur are listed in *Box 3.1*

| Box 3.1 | Where endometriosis is found |
|---|---|
| **Common sites** | **Rarer sites** |
| Ovaries | Pleura |
| Tubes | Lungs |
| Abdominal cavity | Umbilicus |
| Recto-vaginal pouch | Nasal sinuses |
| Uterosacral ligaments | |
| Bowel | |
| Bladder | |
| Cervix | |
| Vagina | |

When it is found in the myometrium it is called adenomyosis

## Presentation

- Dyspareunia. Most commonly due to tender nodules or scarring of the uterosacral ligaments.
- Dysmenorrhoea. Congestive dysmenorrhoea occurs in 25–90% of women with endometriosis. The pain starting most commonly 2–5 days prior to the onset of menstruation although it may be present for up to 2 weeks. The pain usually improves after the first few days of the period and is absent in the follicular phase. It is the cyclical nature of endometriosis which is typical of the condition.
- Abnormal vaginal bleeding occurs in 11–34% of women as IMB, oligomenorrhoea, polymenorrhoea, menorrhagia, post–coital spotting.
- Pain on urinating.
- Cyclical hematuria.
- Pain on defecation.
- Pelvic mass.
- Fixed uterine retroversion.
- Pelvic tenderness.
- Decrease in quality of life.
- Depression.
- Insomnia due to pain.

Symptoms seem to depend on the site rather than the extent and severity of the disease. Twenty-five percent of women with endometriosis are asymptomatic.

In any assessment of the patient it is of paramount importance to assess psychological factors and sexual dysfunction.

Pelvic pain is usually caused by the adhesions that form as a result of the endometrial deposits which bleed in relation to the hormone stimulus (there is no escape for this blood). These adhesions can also distort the pelvic organs and cause dysfunction

The signs and symptoms can be confused with ovarian neoplasm and pelvic inflammatory disease. Women have sometimes presented to their GP many years before they get to see a gynaecologist and have either been tried on unsuccessful treatment, feel that they have not been believed or referred to other specialists due to their presenting symptoms.

## Aetiology

The disease has been linked with:

- increasing age;
- family history;
- heavy periods;
- frequent cycles;
- nulliparous women and women who have never been on the pill.

For this reason it is thought that the increase in the prevalence of this condition is because modern women have fewer children and start their families later in life compared to 50 years ago. Therefore, they have far more menstrual cycles in their lifetime.

## Theories

During menstruation menstrual fluid flows down to the vagina, but there is also reflux back through the fallopian tubes and into the pelvis. It is thought that this reflux causes endometriosis but it is not understood how or why all women do not develop endometriosis. Several theories have been suggested but as yet there is no one theory that has been proved.

- Implantation. It is thought that the menstrual fluid contains viable tissue that implants in the pelvis and then continues to be stimulated by ovarian hormones.
- Coelomic metaplasia. This suggests that peritoneal epithelium changes into endometrial epithelium in response to ovarian hormones.
- Mechanical transplantation. This suggests that endometrium can be transplanted to a different place and implant. This can be seen after uterine surgery where endometriosis has been found in scar tissue on the abdomen.
- Vascular/lymphatic spread. Endometrial tissue can be found in the blood and lymph vessels that drain the uterus. This theory is used to explain the distant spread of endometriosis.
- The COCP and pregnancy protects against endometriosis which supports the theory that it is the cyclical changes in ovarian hormones that supports the development of endometriosis.

## Diagnosis

As well as a full medical and surgical history, the clinician must make a careful evaluation of symptoms; when they first occurred and their relationship with the women's menstrual cycle. This should be followed by a pelvic examination.

Clinicians should utilize ultrasound imaging of the pelvis, when women present with pelvic pain, dysmenorrhoea or dyspareunia to ascertain whether the ovaries are normal or contain endometriotic cysts. The presence of these cysts may indicate more widespread disease in the pelvis. Magnetic resonance imaging may be a useful non-invasive tool in the diagnosis of endometriosis. While it has limitations in the visualization of small endometriotic implants and adhesions, it has the ability to characterize the lesions, to study extraperitoneal locations and the contents of pelvic masses.

The use of serum CA-125 testing has limited value as a screening test for endometriosis. The test's performance in diagnosing all disease stages is limited but for moderate–severe endometriosis was found to be slightly better. Thus, CA-125 has limited value as a screening test or a diagnostic test. It may however, serve as a useful marker for monitoring the effect of treatment once the diagnosis of endometriosis has been established, but again its use has not been evaluated systematically.

The gold standard for the diagnosis of endometriosis is laparoscopy to directly visualize the endometrial deposits. However, diagnostic laparoscopy is associated with 0.06% risk of major complications (e.g. bowel perforation) and this risk is increased to 1.3% in operative laparoscopy.

Endometriosis can resemble blue–black spots, powder burn spots or white plaques on the peritoneum, tubes or ovaries. On the ovaries it normally presents as classic chocolate cysts.

The appearance of endometriosis does not, however, mean that it is this that is causing the symptoms and it can be found coincidentally with other gynaecological conditions. Visual findings need to be accompanied by physical symptoms.

## Endometriosis and fertility

Endometriosis is commonly found in women presenting with subfertility problems. The reason for this link is still unclear.

Thirty to forty percent of women with endometriosis have difficulty conceiving and similarly 30–70% of women investigated for fertility problems are found to have endometriosis.

There is also an increased risk of miscarriage possibly from an inflammatory response in the endometrium and ectopic pregnancy due to reduced tubal motility and/or the distortion of the tubes from adhesions. If the disease is severe and there is damage to structures this will impair fertility, but there is no evidence that the presence of endometriosis causes infertility.

## Treatments

Once a diagnosis of endometriosis had been confirmed there are medical and surgical treatments available.
The aims of the treatment are to:

- relieve pain;
- reduce the size and number of endometriotic deposits;
- restore fertility.

Treatments depend on:

- extent of the disease;
- severity of the disease;
- age of the patient;
- patients desire for future fertility.

### Medical treatments

All medical treatment should be tried for 3 months and then assessed for their effect. If there has been no improvement treatment should be changed. Treatment normally continues for 6 months and is then stopped to assess symptoms. There is a reoccurrence rate of about 15–20%. However, if this is within 6 months of stopping treatment it should be assumed that treatment has failed and another treatment should be tried. Following treatment 50% of women have a reoccurrence within 5 years.

The use of hormonal treatments relies on the principle of stopping/over-riding the woman's menstrual cycle. This can either induce a state of pseudo-pregnancy or pseudomenopause. These two approaches induce atrophy in the ectopic endometrial tissue. The drugs available are equally effective in relieving endometriosis-associated symptoms. However, these drugs are associated with significant side effects that limit their long-term use and often produce poor compliance (*Box 3.2*). In addition, hormonal manipulation probably does not affect any of the primary biological mechanisms responsible for the disease process. Consequently, medical treatment does not always provide complete pain relief and some patients fail to respond.

### Treatment modalities

- NSAIDs are used when patients complain of dysmenorrhoea and are effective with limited side effects. Some women prefer to avoid hormonal therapy and can manage their symptoms effectively with analgesia and/or a complementary medicine approach.

| Box 3.2 | Medical therapies and their side-effects |
| --- | --- |

| Drug | Side effects |
| --- | --- |
| NSAIDS (such as diclofenac, ibuprofen, mefenamic acid) | Gastric irritation |
| Progestogens (such as dydrogesterone, medroxyprogesterone acetate, norethisterone) | Bloating, fluid retention, breast tenderness, nausea |
| Synthetic androgens (such as danazol, gestrinone) | Adverse effects occurred in 15% of women androgenic side effects include acne, weight gain, hirsutism, decreased breast size, muscle cramps, and hunger, seborrhoea, and menopausal symptoms (excluding osteoporosis). The most significant is irreversible voice change. |
| Combined oestrogens and progestogens | Similar to those associated with COCP |
| GnRH analogues (such as buserelin, goserelin, leuprorelin acetate, nafarelin, triptorelin) | Menopausal symptoms (including osteoporosis) |
| GnRH analogues and any combined hormone replacement therapy (continuous or sequential) or tibolone | Adverse effects occur in 11% of women taking GnRH analogues, which are associated with hypo-oestrogenic symptoms such as hot flushes and vaginal dryness. Adding hormone replacement therapy ameliorates the side effects of GnRH analogues |

- Progestogens. High dose progestogens can give relief in about 70–80% of patients. They do, however, have side effects that patients can find intolerable such as weight gain, breast tenderness and breakthrough bleeding.
- Danazol. Can give relief in 90% of patients but the side effects mean that about 20% of patients will discontinue treatment. Clinical trials and scientific experiments have shown Danazol to be the most effective treatment since it seems to act by reducing the inflammatory response as well as having a hormonal effect.
- COCP. If a woman is not trying to conceive and there is no evidence of a pelvic mass on examination, there may be a role for a therapeutic trial of a COCP (monthly or tricycling) or a progestogen to treat pain symptoms suggestive of endometriosis without performing a diagnostic laparoscopy first. This treatment can also be used after a diagnosis of endometriosis.
- Gonadotrophin releasing hormone (GnRH) analogues. These suppress LH and FSH secretion in the pituitary so there is no ovarian function and the endometriosis shrinks. This can give relief in about 90% of patients and the side effects can be reduced by giving add back therapy in the form of Tibolone.

The choice between the COCP, progestogens, danazol and GnRH agonists depends principally upon their side-effect profiles because they relieve pain associated with endometriosis equally well.

Duration of therapy is limited for some drugs due to the side-effect profile. The COCP and Depo-Provera may be used long-term, but the use of gestogens, danazol and GnRH agonists is usually restricted to 6 months. GnRH agonist therapy is limited because up to 6% of bone mineral density may be lost in the first 6 months. However, the loss is restored almost completely 2 years after stopping treatment. 'Add-back' therapy (i.e. progestogen with or without oestrogen) can be used to relieve menopausal side effects, to prevent bone loss and allow therapy to continue beyond 6 months. How long this regimen may safely be continued is unclear. Lastly, there is some evidence to suggest that GnRH agonist treatment for 3 months may be as effective as 6 months' treatment.

### Surgical treatments

- Laporoscopy and diathermy to the endometriosis.
- Laparoscopy and ovarian cystectomy. There is some evidence that pain and subfertility caused by ovarian endometrioma is improved more by cystectomy than by simple cyst drainage and cautery.
- Laporotomy and reconstructive surgery.
- Hysterectomy with removal of both ovaries. Cure will only be achieved by removing both ovaries so this treatment should ideally only be offered to women in their late thirties or early forties who have completed their families.

Laparoscopic ablation of minimal–moderate endometriosis appears to relieve pain, although it is unclear whether uterine nerve ablation is required as well.

Surgery can be used separately although more commonly medical treatments are used after surgical procedures to enhance and prolong the symptom-free period. Six months' postoperative treatment with GnRH analogues or a combination of danazol and medroxyprogesterone can significantly reduce pain and delay the recurrence of pain.

### Supportive therapies

Patients increasingly want information about complimentary therapies. These can be of some value in helping the women to cope with her symptoms. Some women have found benefit from taking vitamins, minerals and herbal medicine. There is no doubt that a consultation in which the severity of the woman's symptoms is believed can be of enormous benefit. Women with endometriosis have often been trying to get help for their symptoms for a long time and may have been misdiagnosed or simply not believed. There is a strong role for a therapeutic consultation particularly from nursing staff with discussion about coping strategies for pain management. Women who have had symptoms for a long time often have low self-esteem and may find acupuncture, massage and reflexology extremely helpful. They may benefit from joining a support group for patients with endometriosis.

## Endometriosis and cancer

As yet there is no evidence of a direct link between endometriosis and cancer. There is some suggestion that malignancies are more commonly found in ovaries that contain endometriosis. Clear cell and endometroid carcinomas are most commonly seen in endometriotic ovaries and there is a clear association between these histological types and endometriosis. Clinicians and patients must be made aware of this association especially when surgery is contemplated in relatively young women.

# Premenstrual syndrome (PMS)

The existence of PMS as a distinct clinical entity remains controversial. The term premenstrual tension (PMT) was first used by Frank in 1931 who described tension, depression, weight gain and headaches in women 7–10 days prior to the onset of menstruation. Green and Dalton first used the term PMS in 1953. More recently the American Psychiatric Society has renamed the syndrome late luteal phase dysphonic disorder.

## Prevalence

It is estimated that PMS affects about 1.5 million women to such an extent that that their quality of life and interpersonal relationships can be affected. It affects women irrespective of socio-economic status, race and cultural background.

It has been estimated that 90% of women are aware of changes in themselves in the menstrual cycle. It is, however, only a small minority that suffer so severely that they come to the attention of the medical profession. About 40% of women experience some of the symptoms of PMS but only 5–10% of women have symptoms that significantly interfere with their ability to live a normal life.

## Definition

PMS can be defined as the recurrence of psychological and physical symptoms in the luteal phase, which remit in follicular phase of the menstrual cycle.

It is therefore the characteristic cyclical nature of the symptoms and not the symptoms themselves that make the diagnosis of PMS. The severity of the symptoms can fluctuate from cycle to cycle but the type of symptoms remains constant in each individual.

PMS seems to be less severe at menarche but becomes more severe throughout the reproductive years before merging with the symptoms of the climacteric. The symptoms can start at ovulation and progress through to the menstrual cycle. It therefore follows that if the woman has a short menstrual cycle she can have very few symptom-free days each month.

There are also 160 medical conditions that can fluctuate with each cycle. These include asthma, epilepsy, migraine, RA and herpes. A careful history taking should reveal any of these as an underlying cause that needs treatment.

## Evaluation of PMS

### History

- Type of symptoms positive and negative.
- When the symptoms started – linkage to COCP and/or pregnancy.
- Relationship to the cycle.
- Resolution in relation to menses.
- A full menstrual history.
- Contraceptive history.
- Obstetric history.
- Gynaecological history.
- Medical history.
- Surgical history.
- Psychiatric and psychological history.
- Social history, particularly regarding work and relationships with partner/children/family.

### Physical examination

It is important to get the patient to list all her symptoms and grade them according to their severity. A menstrual distress questionnaire can be used but there is no validated and widely accepted rating scale for PMS. The patient must keep a diary of the most severe symptoms, noting timing, frequency and severity using a visual analogue or numerical score.

## Signs and symptoms

### Physical

- Breast tenderness and swelling.
- Abdominal bloating.
- Peripheral oedema.
- Headaches/ migraines.
- Hot flushes.
- Dizziness.
- Palpitations.

- Visual disturbances.
- Pelvic discomfort.
- Altered bowel habits.
- Appetite changes/cravings.
- Nausea.
- Acne.
- Decrease in co-ordination.
- Bloating and fluid retention give the impression of weight gain but no demonstrable weight gain.

## Psychological

- Tension.
- Irritability.
- Depression.
- Mood swings.
- Anxiety.
- Restlessness.
- Lethargy.
- Decreased libido.

## Behavioural

- Agoraphobia.
- Absenteeism from work.
- Decreased concentration.
- Decreased work performance.
- Avoidance of social activities.
- Increase in accidents.
- Increase in alcoholic binges.
- Increase in criminal behaviours.
- Increase in suicide attempts.

However, 5–15% of women actually feel better premenstrually and even report an increase in libido.

## Investigation

There are multiple theories to try and explain the underlying pathophysiology of PMS. None of them have been proved scientifically or led to highly successful therapies. These include the following:

- progesterone deficit;
- oestrogen/progesterone imbalance;

- sodium and water retention;
- prostaglandin deficit/excess;
- prolactin excess;
- vitamin B6 deficit;
- trace element deficit;
- hypoglycaemia;
- thyroid abnormality;
- serotonin deficit;
- neurotransmitters;
- psychological;
- diet;
- drugs;
- lifestyle.

Diagnostic investigations have tried to detect abnormalities that could reflect these theories but usually all come back as normal. There is, therefore, no objective way to diagnose PMS. Hormone tests, including a full blood count to rule out anaemia and thyroid function tests to rule out hypothyroidism, are not reliable but can be useful in excluding other diseases that can produce similar symptoms. A reproductive hormone profile may detect the climacteric or poly-cystic ovaries (PCOS) although there is no evidence that PCOS is associated with an increased prevalence of PMS. However, women suffering from PCOS do need health advice about maintaining a stable weight to prevent late-onset diabetes, hirsutism and oligoamenorrhoea.

## Treatment

It is important to remember to treat the woman with PMS and not the PMS itself. There needs to be a holistic management plan for the syndrome and not a symptom/disease management plan. It is important to recognize that initial discussion and subsequent counselling has a therapeutic effect that is often more important than any more physical therapy. Acknowledgment that the severity of the symptoms causes disruption to her life is important. The discussion needs to include advice on diet, stress awareness and lifestyle and is an opportunity to increase knowledge and understanding of the menstrual cycle. It is also essential to establish realistic expectations for the outcome of treatment.

It has been noted that there is a high placebo response rate especially to psychological rather than physical symptoms.

Medical therapies

- Selective serotonin reuptake inhibitors: Fluoxetine has been shown to be one of the most effective treatments.

- Diuretics: spironolactone.
- Prostaglandin inhibitors: ponstan taken from day 16 of the cycle.
- Buspirone.
- Aliprazolam.
- Tranquillizers/antidepressants.
- Bromocriptine for breast pain.
- Progesterone: although there is no evidence of its effectiveness but it is often first line treatment.
- Suppression of the ovarian cycle:
  (a) COCP: this can be effective, however if taken cyclically then the patient may get symptoms in the pill-free week. It should be the first line treatment if the women need contraceptive cover and can be tricycled to minimize symptom return in the pill-free week.
  (b) If symptoms are still present try and change to a different progestogen.
- Danazol: this suppresses ovulation and can be beneficial if the patient complains of severe mastalgia. It does have androgenic effects and cannot be used long term. There is a suggestion that it may be beneficial at lower doses and used in the luteal phase only.
- GnRH analogues: these have been proven to be more effective than placebo but can again only be used for short-term relief due to the adverse effect on bone density. There is some evidence to suggest that symptoms return with add back HRT. They can be used diagnostically in finding out if the symptoms are true PMS and not psychological.
- Oestrogen: given either as an implant or transdermally. The dose needed is higher than in HRT, 100–200 μg patches being given with progesterone for 10 days every 3 months to protect the endometrium. This can cause a recurrence of symptoms. The progestogen releasing IUS can be used instead of cyclical progestogen to good effect although there is no long-term data on whether the endometrium is fully protected.
- TAH BSO – a final option.

## Self-help groups

Patients can find it very therapeutic to talk to other women who suffer from the same problems and can gain reassurance that they are not going mad. These groups can be founded by a motivated patient or by a nurse with an interest in PMS. Once established the facilitator should be able to take a back seat and involve the patients in the running of the group. It is important that a suitable venue is found which is easily accessible for the women and not too clinical an environment.

## General self-help measures

- Diet: will not have immediate effects.

- Eat well: general health promotion:
  (a) Reduce: salt; fluid intake; caffeine; fat; junk foods; alcohol and tobacco.
  (b) Increase: calcium; vitamin E; magnesium; potassium.
- Eat regularly.
- Do not over eat.
- Increase exercise.
- Increase relaxation.

All of these measures will improve health and self-esteem.
Additional life style measures include:

- stress management;
- arrange breaks from childcare;
- avoid stressful social situations.

Nutritional supplements of vitamin B6 can be helpful since it is a co factor in neurotransmitter synthesis. Evening primrose oil can be useful for breast pain.

### Alternative therapies

Many women use alternative and complimentary therapies rather than conventional medical treatment. If women wish to persue this line of treatment it is advisable that they consult a recognized practitioner.

There has been some success in treatment of PMS with homeopathy, chiropractic therapy and herbal treatments such as Vitex Angus Chaste.

## Summary

PMS can affect all women. For some their symptoms can be severely debilitating and affect the quality of life and ability to function normally at home, work or in social situations. After ruling out any underlying disease treatment should be holistic, supportive and aimed at resolving or minimizing the presenting symptoms.

# 4 Reproductive Medicine and Subfertility

## Oligomenorrhoea and secondary amenorrhoea

The principal anxiety of women referred with irregular periods or an absence of periods for greater than 6 months is their future fertility. A proportion will present with hirsutism together with oligoamenorrhoea. In order to speed up the time to diagnosis and treatment interval these women can have their initial investigations performed by their GP. The outpatient appointment should be sent with a request for a pregnancy test, luteinizing hormone (LH), follicle stimulating hormone (FSH), testosterone (T), prolactin (PRL), oestradiol (E2) and a transvaginal ultrasound scan (*Box 4.1*). Since these women do not cycle regularly there is no point in waiting for the next period in order to do the tests. If the GP has started the woman on oral contraception then this should be stopped for at least 1 month prior to testing and barrier contraception methods advised.

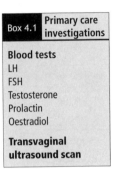

| Box 4.1 | Primary care investigations |
|---|---|
| **Blood tests** | |
| LH | |
| FSH | |
| Testosterone | |
| Prolactin | |
| Oestradiol | |
| **Transvaginal ultrasound scan** | |

### Definitions

- Oligomenorrhoea: cycle length of greater than 35 days or fewer than five menses per year.
- Secondary amenorrhoea: no periods for more than 6 months or a three-fold change in cycle length.

### Differential diagnoses (see *Figure 4.1*)

- Pregnancy. This remains the commonest cause of secondary amenorrhoea and women with oligomenorrhoea may be pregnant unexpectedly since they are often advised that they are unable to have children and, therefore, do not use adequate contraception.
- PCOS. This syndrome occurs in 1:4 women and may present in many different ways. Eighty five percent of women with oligomenorrhoea and 32% of women with secondary amenorrhoea will have PCOS as their underlying diagnosis.
- Hypogonadotrophic hypogonadism (HH). The commonest cause is weight related (anorexia, bulimia) or excessive exercise (gymnasts, ballerinas, long distance runners). Sometimes it is due to a delay in hypothalamic recovery from depot contraceptive methods.

- Hyperprolactinaemia. Presents with secondary amenorrhoea or occasionally oligomenorrhoea sometimes associated with galactorrhoea. It is most often due to a micro- or macroadenoma. Although 20% of women with PCOS have a raised prolactin it is not the primary cause of their oligoamenorrhoea unless the prolactin level is >1000.
- Premature ovarian failure. This condition affects 1% of women under the age of 30 and 3% of women under the age of 40. It is rarely associated with fragile X syndrome or autoimmune multiple endocrinopathy syndrome. FSH receptor abnormalities and metabolic problems.
- Asherman's syndrome. These women present with secondary amenorrhoea most commonly following repeated evacuation of retained products following pregnancy, termination of pregnancy or routine dilatation and curettage, transcervical resection of the endometrium or submucosal fibroids.

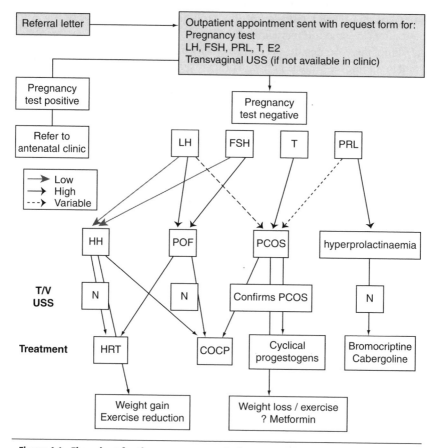

Figure 4.1. Flow chart for the management of oligoamenorrhoea

# Evaluation

A careful history can accurately narrow down the differential diagnosis amongst the majority of women. All women should be asked the details shown in *Box 4.2*. Particular attention needs to be paid to changes in cycle length that may be secondary to changes in weight and lifestyle. Physical examination will not add greatly to achieving a diagnosis although it is worth examining for galactorrhoea, visual field abnormalities, acne and hirsutism.

| Box 4.2 History | | | |
|---|---|---|---|
| **Menstrual cycle** | **Associated symptoms** | **Family history** | **Past medical/ social history** |
| Cycle length | Acne/hirsutism | Oligoamenorrhoea | Anorexia/bulimia |
| Menarche | Galactorrhoea | Type 2 diabetes | Contraceptive |
| Duration of | Weight change | Hirsutism/acne | history |
| symptoms | Exercise pattern | Fragile X syndrome | Past obstetric |
| Previous cycle | Subfertility | (male) | history |
| length | Nausea/breast | Recurrent miscarriage | |
| Blood loss | tenderness | | |

- Pregnancy is diagnosed by a simple urine test that detects hCG. All gynaecological clinics should have a means of rapidly doing hCG tests.
- PCOS. The diagnosis depends on both endocrinological and ultrasound findings. A raised testosterone ($>2.4 < 5$ nmol/l) is the commonest and most diagnostic endocrine test (85% of cases) with a raised LH ($>10.1$ IU/l) found in between 45% and 70% of cases. An ultrasound scan is the most diagnostic and it is important that ultrasonographers are trained in the criteria for PCOS (*Figure 4.2*). These include two out of the following three morphological findings:
  (1) more than 10 follicles of less than 10 mm in a single cross-section of the ovary;
  (2) an increased stromal density and/or increased stromal volume;
  (3) an ovarian volume of $> 9$ cm$^3$.
- HH. The diagnosis of this condition depends on careful history taking of weight change, exercise undertaken and recent contraceptive methods. The diagnosis is made through accurate determination of weight and height to calculate Body Mass Index (BMI= wt in kg/height in m$^2$). The hormone profile usually shows a low LH, FSH and E2 with normal prolactin and testosterone. The ultrasound will be essentially normal although occasionally multi-follicular ovaries are present. This is often a sign of recovering HH and can be associated with normal LH and FSH. Multi-follicular ovaries are those

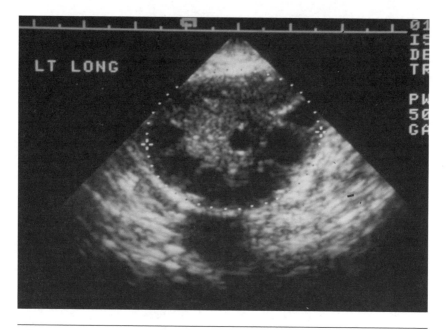

**Figure 4.2. Ultrasound of a polycystic ovary**

with >6 but <10 follicles in a single cross-section with a normal stromal density and volume.

- Hyperprolactinaemia. This is diagnosed with a raised prolactin level of >1000 IU/l. At levels below 2500 IU/l it is unusual for a macroadenoma to be present but all patients should have a CT scan of the pituitary and a visual field test. The LH, FSH and E2 will usually be low with a normal testosterone.
- Premature ovarian failure. This condition is characterized by a raised FSH (>12 IU/l) on two occasions. It is a distressing condition because no treatment has been found that restores fertility. Careful counselling is required and many of these women need formal counselling and support to come to terms with their lack of fertility options. Additional investigations should include genetic analysis at a regional center for fragile X and an autoimmune screen for anti-thyroid, anti-adrenal and anti-ovarian antibodies.
- Asherman's syndrome. The hormone profile is normal in these women but the ultrasound scan can show a thin, brightly echogenic endometrium or an endometrium with multiple cystic spaces where small islands of endometrium are still active but the synechiae within the uterus are trapping the small amounts of menstrual blood within the cavity.

The use of a progesterone withdrawal test (Medroxyprogesterone acetate 10 mg/day for 5 days) will identify those women with naturally circulating oestrogen and is an additional test for PCOS which is of limited diagnostic use.

## Treatment

**Pregnancy.** Refer for an ultrasound for accurate dating and arrange antenatal care.

**PCOS.** The treatment depends on the needs of the woman. If she wishes to become pregnant and has been trying for over 1 year and is in a stable relationship refer her to the subfertility clinic. If her principal concern is lack of periods and contraception is required and she has no contraindications then COCP is the treatment of choice since it will induce regular periods and reduce the risk of endometrial hyperplasia and dysfunctional uterine bleeding. The pills of choice are dianette as it contains an anti-androgen and may help acne and hirsutism, and marvelon or femodene as these contain less androgenic progestogens than some of the first and second generation COCPs. If the patient has contraindications for the COCP then regular withdrawal bleeds (at least every 3 months) can be induced by giving a progestogen for 10 days (medroxy-progesterone acetate or duphaston 10 mg o.d).

Women with PCOS who are significantly overweight (BMI $> 28$ kg/m$^2$) should be encouraged to lose weight. Some women will be able to tell you what weight they were when their periods became irregular and they should aim for this weight since it is highly likely that their periods will become more regular and improve any acne or hirsutism they have. The use of metformin without a reduction in calorie intake will not have a long-lasting effect and can be associated with significant gastro-intestinal side effects. Women with PCOS are poor energy consumers and so need to have a diet of less than 1200 calories per day to have a good chance of losing weight. The targets should be realistically small for each time interval with a maximum goal of 5 kg per 3 months.

Hirsutism is difficult to treat. No medication will cure it and the problem will return when medication is stopped. Combined with oligomenorrhoea dianette is ideal since it contains oestrogen and the anti-androgen cyproterone acetate. If after 3 months there has been no reduction in the rate of growth of the hair then additional cyproterone acetate, 50 mg, can be added for the first 10 days of each packet. This can be safely continued for 1 year when the maximum benefit will have been achieved and the situation maintained on dianette alone. Dianette should be continued until the woman wants fertility. If the woman is not able to take the COCP then she can be offered spironolactone 100 mg OD continuously. Again, the maximum effect of reduction in rate of hair growth will be achieved by 6 months to 1 year. Increasing the dose does not seem to make a difference.

**HH.** Similar to PCOS the treatment depends on the needs of the woman. If she wishes to become pregnant and has been trying for over 1 year and is in a stable relationship refer her to the subfertility clinic. If her principal concern is lack of periods and contraception is required and she has no contraindications then the COCP is the treatment of choice since it will induce regular periods and provide oestrogen to prevent hypooestrogenic osteoporosis.

**Hyperprolactinaemia.** The treatment of choice is a dopamine agonist such as bromocriptine or cabergoline. These need to be started at a low dose and then increased according to the level of prolactin until normal levels are reached. The prolactin should be checked every 4 weeks until the levels normalize and/or the woman's periods restart. Once a steady state is reached the prolactin levels can be checked annually unless the woman becomes amenorrhoeic. The oral contraceptive pill should not be used so these women should be advised to use barrier methods or an intrauterine contraceptive device if they do not wish to become pregnant.

**Premature ovarian failure.** These women require HRT using the oral contraceptive pill or conventional HRT.

**Asherman's syndrome.** A hysteroscopy should be performed with division of the synechiae. An IUCD should be inserted at the end of the procedure and the patient should be started on high dose oestrogen patches to encourage the endometrium to grow over the scarred areas. After 3 months an ultrasound should be repeated to confirm a regular, smooth endometrium and the IUCD removed.

## Primary amenorrhoea

Primary amenorrhoea is a much rarer condition than secondary amenorrhoea. The need to investigate the condition depends on the presence or absence of secondary sexual characteristics. Many of the causes of primary amenorrhoea may have profound implications for the teenager and her family since many preclude the possibility of childbearing. It is therefore important to bear this in mind before commencing on invasive and complicated investigations that may in themselves cause distress to a young woman who is already anxious because she is not the same as her peers. Their mothers, and/or fathers and occasionally grandparents accompany nearly all these young girls. These adults are usually very concerned and may unintentionally increase the distress of the child. It is therefore essential that an assessment of how aware the child may be of why she has been referred should be made. If necessary the parents need to be seen separately from the child with clear explanations of the investigations and what they may uncover prior to proceeding with testing particularly when it is invasive. Teenagers vary enormously in how much they can understand and sensitivity is required to make sure that the information they receive is easy to understand and pertinent to their stage of psychological and emotional as well as physical development. Easy and prompt access to a counsellor is strongly recommended.

## Definitions

- The absence of menstruation by the age of 14 in the absence of growth or development of secondary sexual characteristics.
- The absence of menstruation by the age of 16 despite normal growth and development of secondary sexual characteristics.

## Differential diagnosis

### Chromosomal

- Turner's syndrome. Ovarian dysgenesis secondary to the absence of one X-chromosome, karyotype 45 XO. Mosaics or deletions in the long or short arms of the X chromosome may occur in up to 25% of cases.
- Androgen insensitivity syndrome (AIS). Complete or partial deletion in the androgen receptor gene on the Y chromosome. This leads to regression of the mullerian system so the upper two-thirds of the vagina, the uterus and fallopian tubes are absent, and the testes are usually in the inguinal canal but may be found in the abdomen or labia majora. The external genitalia are usually of normal female phenotype but there may be partial virilization in some patients. The karyotype is XY.

### Anatomical

- Cryptomenorrhoea. This is most commonly due to an imperforate hymen but may be due to a blockage higher up in the genital tract.
- Mullerian agenesis. Failure of the mullerian duct to develop, this is rarely a complete defect and may involve failure of the upper vagina to develop with a normal uterus and fallopian tubes but there may be an absence of the uterus.
- Kallman's syndrome. The association of amenorrhoea with anosmia secondary to the failure of development of the olfactory plate and the hypothalamus in fetal life.

### Acquired

- Infection in early gestation may lead to gonadal dysgenesis.
- Chemotherapy or radiotherapy in childhood for the treatment of childhood malignancies, particularly leukaemia and lymphoma.
- Hypothalamic/pituitary surgery in childhood for craniopharyngioma.

# Evaluation

A careful history and sensitive examination may lead to the diagnosis but needs to be confirmed by investigations. In primary amenorrhoea the symptoms may backdate to infancy but their importance may not have been understood at the time. The investigations are similar to oligoamenorrhoea with the addition of karyotyping

- Turner's syndrome. Women with Turner's syndrome may have any or all of the following features.
  (a) History:
    (1) slow at school;
    (2) poor growth/failure to thrive in infancy;
    (3) no periods.
  (b) Examination:
    (1) short stature;
    (2) webbed neck;
    (3) wide carrying angle.
- AIS. Women with partial AIS have often been diagnosed in infancy because of clitoromegaly or removal of the gonads because of inguinal hernias. Unfortunately the diagnosis is often not explained to these girls, surgery may have been undertaken without their consent and therefore they may distrust doctors. Establishing a good relationship with them and listening to their principle concerns with good explanations can markedly reduce some of the psychological stigmata these women often suffer. The results of investigation will depend on whether a gonadectomy has been performed.
  (a) History:
    (1) clitoromegaly;
    (2) hernia repairs in childhood;
    (3) difficulty with intercourse;
    (4) normal mental development;
    (5) normal height.
  (b) Examination:
    (1) variable breast development;
    (2) absent/sparse pubic/axillary hair;
    (3) surgical scarring/ absent or short vagina.
- Cryptomenorrhoea.
  (a) History:
    (1) cyclical dysmenorrhoea;
    (2) pressure symptoms.
  (b) Examination:
    (1) bluish, bulging membrane at introitus;
    (2) thick transverse membrane across vagina;
    (3) abdominal mass.

- Mullerian agenesis. The main history is absence of periods with normal breast development and pubic/ axillary hair growth. On examination there is a blind ending vagina or shortened vagina.
- General questions to ask. Infections in childhood; operations in childhood/early adolescence; sense of smell; childhood tumours and subsequent therapy.

## Investigations and their interpretation

The investigations required include a full hormone profile, a karyotype and in those where a significant mullerian defect is suspected, a laparoscopy should be performed. *Table 4.1* shows an easy way to interpret the results and arrive at a diagnosis.

**Table 4.1.** Differential diagnosis of primary amenorrhoea

| Diagnosis | LH | FSH | Testosterone | Oestradiol | Karyotype |
|---|---|---|---|---|---|
| Turners syndrome | High | High | Normal | Low | 45 XO (or mosaic) |
| AIS | High | High/ normal | Male range or low | Low | 46 XY |
| **Anatomical** Genital tract anomaly | Normal | Normal | Normal | Normal | Normal |
| Hypothalamic anomaly | Low | Low | Low/normal | Low | Normal |
| **Childhood tumours** Intrathecal CT or cranial DXT | Low | Low | Low/normal | Low | Normal |
| Chemotherapy/ abdominopelvic DXT | High | High | Low/normal | Low | Normal |

## Treatment

The choice of treatment depends on the needs of the woman. In some of the conditions fertility will not be possible, in others egg donation or surrogacy may be an option. The latter has significant problems. Referral to an Assisted Conception Unit is advised and for those for whom fertility is not possible or where there are difficulties in coming to terms with the implications of the condition referral to specialist counselling services, support groups and tertiary referral centers specializing in the rarer conditions is recommended.

### Surgery

- Cryptomenorrhoea can usually be treated simply and effectively with a cruciate incision of the hymen and oversewing of the edges.
- Thickened vaginal septae, complex mullerian tract anomalies, particularly if they are associated with renal anomalies, should be referred to specialist centres.

### Oestrogen replacement therapy

All these groups of women require hormone replacement therapy with the exception of the anatomical anomalies that require surgery. Some of the women with AIS may need testosterone replacement as well as or instead of oestrogen replacement.

# Subfertility

Difficulty in conceiving is one of the commonest reasons for referral to the gynaecology clinic. Ideally a team who specializes in subfertility should run the clinic. There should also be arrangements for serial scanning, ovulation induction, intrauterine insemination and assisted conception and ready access to members of the team if problems are encountered or results are needed during the course of treatment.

## Referral

Criteria for referral to the subfertility clinic must be quite strict and should be vetted by a senior member of the subfertility team prior to the appointment being sent. Our criteria are:

- difficulty conceiving for more than 1 year with the same partner;
- the couple should have been in a stable relationship for greater than 2 years.

When the appointment is sent out a letter is enclosed requesting that the patient goes to their GP and makes arrangements for the initial investigations (*Box 4.3*). The letter should clearly state that the patient will not have any further investigations performed or be offered any treatment unless all the results are available at the first appointment. It should be explained that without all the results it is not possible to advise the couple on the correct mode of treatment for them and therefore unsafe to offer treatment.

## First visit

A full history and examination of both partners should be taken. The results of the hormone profile, rubella screen, mid-luteal progesterone and male fertility tests should be reviewed in order to establish the most likely underlying abnormality.

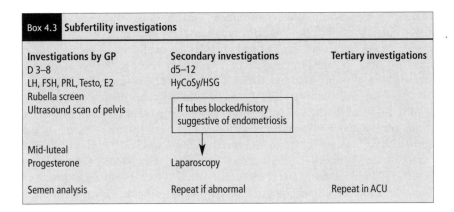

| Box 4.3 | Subfertility investigations | | |
|---|---|---|---|
| **Investigations by GP** | **Secondary investigations** | **Tertiary investigations** | |
| D 3–8 | d5–12 | | |
| LH, FSH, PRL, Testo, E2 | HyCoSy/HSG | | |
| Rubella screen | | | |
| Ultrasound scan of pelvis | If tubes blocked/history suggestive of endometriosis | | |
| Mid-luteal | ↓ | | |
| Progesterone | Laparoscopy | | |
| Semen analysis | Repeat if abnormal | Repeat in ACU | |

The results should be explained clearly to the couple (see *Box 4.4* for normal values). The diagnoses should fit into one of three categories: anovulation; male fertility problem; tubal disease. With advancing techniques of examining a semen sample the percentage of couples with underlying male subfertility has risen and the number of couples with truly unexplained subfertility has reduced.

| Box 4.4 | Normal values | | |
|---|---|---|---|
| **Hormone profile d5–8** | | **Semen analysis** | |
| LH | 3–10 IU/l | Count | >40 million/ml |
| FSH | 3–9.9 IU/l | Volume | 2–5 ml |
| Prolactin | <480 IU/l | Motility | >50% progressively motile |
| Testosterone | 0.9–2.4 nmol/l | Morphology | <30% abnormal |
| **Mid-luteal progesterone >30 nmol/l** | | | |

Anovulation may be associated with primary or secondary amenorrhoea. However, very irregular menses (cycle length greater than 42 days) significantly reduce the chances of becoming pregnant not because of the difficulty in predicting the day of ovulation but because the number of eggs produced per annum are reduced. Compare the following, a 28 day cycle means that 13 eggs are produced each year whilst a 42 day cycle reduces this to 8, and a 56 day cycle to 6 etc. The commonest cause of this pattern is PCOS which usually responds to weight loss and/or clomiphene.

Male fertility problems may be associated with chromosomal abnormalities (e.g. Kleinfelter's syndrome), hormonal (hypogonadotrophic hypogonadism, premature testicular failure) or structural problems (absent vas deferens, epididimal cysts, hydrocoele). In all these cases the client should be referred to an andrologist or urologist. More commonly low sperm counts and/or low motility may be associated with some environmental factors such as smoking (particularly cannabis), alcohol and certain occupations (classically long distance drivers, chefs, non-ground based airline personnel). Occasionally the abnormality may be transient as in recent or concurrent illnesses, incorrect collection of sample, long delay from production to analysis. The majority however are unexplained.

Repeating any abnormal tests is worthwhile and reassuring for the couple. Whilst these are being repeated investigations for tubal patency should be arranged. HyCoSy investigation is performed using ultrasound (*Figure 4.4*). A small catheter is passed through the cervix and a special fluid that is easily visible on ultrasound is injected. The fluid can be seen travelling along the tubes and into the abdominal cavity. In the event of a cornual block or a hydrosalpinx then it is worth further investigating the block with a formal hysterosalpingogram (*Figure 4.5*). Ideally both should be available at the same time. It is possible to divide women into high and low risk categories for tubal block from their history and initial ultrasound scan (a hydrosalpinx may have been seen). The low risk group can be offered HyCoSy alone whilst high-risk women should have a HSG as well. These investigations identify uterine anomalies such as endometrial polyps, submucosal fibroids or bicornuate uteri and significant septa.

The passage of the catheter into the cervix is associated with a risk of pelvic infection and therefore it is wise to offer prophylaxis with a single PR dose of Metronidazole and a 5-day course of Doxycycline 100 mg bd. The procedure

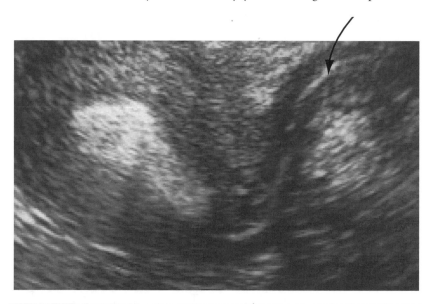

**Figure 4.4. Hysterocontrastsalpingosonography (HyCoSy). The arrow indicates the lumen of the fallopian tube.**

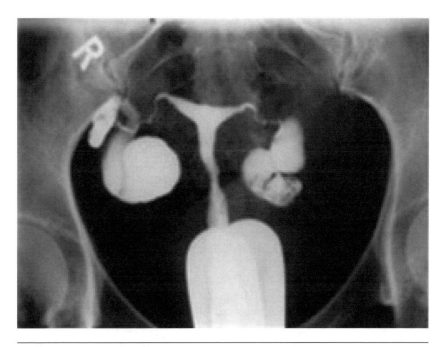

**Figure 4.5. Hysterosalpingogram showing bilateral hydrosalpinges**

itself can be painful so the offer of pain relief 1 hour prior to the procedure is advised.

## Second visit

The second visit should be an opportunity to review the results and make a diagnosis. The relevant treatment options can then be discussed with the couple. Unhappily most health authorities do not fund subfertility treatments except clomiphene therapy. A few will fund a single cycle of assisted conception and /or intrauterine insemination (IUI). The treatment options are outlined in *Box 4.5*.

Each option requires careful organization to ensure that the risks of subfertility treatment are minimized. The professional team and their roles are illustrated in *Box 4.6*.

### Treatment

**Anovulation clomiphene.** If the patient has PCOS and has a BMI of less than 30 kg/m$^2$ then the woman should be prescribed clomiphene 50 mg once a day from day 3–7 inclusive of the cycle. If the cycle length is very irregular then she should

## Box 4.5 Treatment options

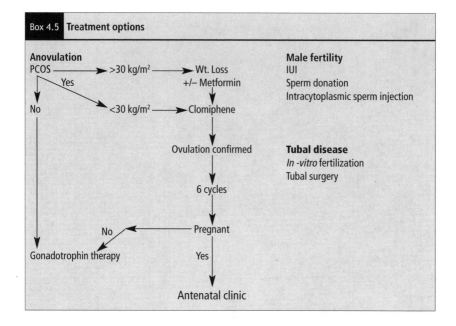

**Anovulation**

PCOS ──→ >30 kg/m² ──→ Wt. Loss
      Yes              +/– Metformin

No ──→ <30 kg/m² ──→ Clomiphene

Ovulation confirmed

6 cycles

No ←── Pregnant

Gonadotrophin therapy       Yes

Antenatal clinic

**Male fertility**
IUI
Sperm donation
Intracytoplasmic sperm injection

**Tubal disease**
*In -vitro* fertilization
Tubal surgery

take a progestogen (e.g. Medroxyprogesterone acetate 10 mg o.d) for 10 days in order to produce a withdrawal bleed. If there is no withdrawal bleed then the woman can start the clomiphene on the 7th day after completing the progestogen and call that day 3. It is essential to start at 50 mg clomiphene to minimize the risk

## Box 4.6 The team

| | |
|---|---|
| Clerk/receptionist | Making appointments, tracing and preparing files |
| Secretary | Letter writing, answering queries, liaison within team |
| Nursing staff | History taking, liaising with patient and GP<br>Education and counselling of couple<br>Training woman or partner to give injections<br>Treatment monitoring and advice |
| Medical staff | HyCoSy/HSG<br>History and examination. Initiation of treatment |
| Ultrasonographer<br>(if nursing and medical staff not trained) | Diagnostic tests, uterine anomalies, ovarian morphology<br>Follicular tracking |
| Cytologist/embryologist | Semen analysis<br>Sperm preparation for IUI |

of multiple pregnancy (10%) and ovarian hyperstimulation syndrome (2%). In order to confirm ovulation a progesterone level should be taken on day 21 and again on day 24. The couple should be given a contact number so that they can obtain the result of the test prior to the expected onset of menses. If the result demonstrates ovulation and the woman has a period then she can repeat the treatment a further five times. If she fails to have a period then she should perform a pregnancy test.

If she fails to ovulate then the dose of clomiphene can be increased to 100 mg o.d. from day 3–7 with a repeat progesterone test. If she fails to ovulate at this dose then the dose can be increased to 150 mg o.d. from day 3 to 7 on the same regimen as before. If the treatment fails at this dose then ovulation induction with gonadotrophins should be offered since no benefit is gained at higher doses.

For those women with PCOS whose BMI is greater than 30 kg/m² weight loss is the best option since this increases the chances of achieving ovulation and reduces the risk of miscarriage. Women with PCOS find losing weight harder than other women because of their insulin resistance. They require a great deal of support and special support groups run by fitness instructors and dieticians have been found to be the most useful in helping these women. Metformin (500 mg tds) can be used in addition to a low calorie diet (1200 kcal/day). Once weight loss of > 5% of starting weight or a decrease in clothes size is noted then clomiphene can be started.

**Gonadotrophin therapy.** The gonadotrophin used to induce ovulation is FSH. It can be used for all women who fail to ovulate and have no other fertility problems except those with premature ovarian failure or chromosomal abnormalities. The administration of this treatment is by intramuscular or subcutaneous injection. The woman, her partner or her GP's surgery can administrate the injections. Subcutaneous administration is the easiest for the woman to learn. Ultrasound monitoring of follicular development is essential in order to ensure that no more than three follicles reach maturity (*Figure 4.6*) and to decide when to give human chorionic gonadotrophin to release the ova when the follicle has reached 18–20 mm in diameter.

In women with PCOS who are at increased risk of multiple follicular development the dose of gonadotrophin should commence in every cycle at 75 IU per day or less. In the first cycle this should continue for 14 days before increasing to 112.5 IU for a further 7 days if no dominant follicle (12 mm in diameter). Seventy five percent of women will develop a dominant follicle at this dose and 85% at 150 IU/day. Using this regimen less than 1% of women will develop more than three follicles and the risk of ovarian hyperstimulation is minimal.

**Male fertility.** The treatment of choice for men with oligospermia depends on the degree of oligospermia and the motility of the sperm. If adequate numbers of sperm ($>1 \times 10^6$ motile sperm/ml) can be prepared by the laboratory staff

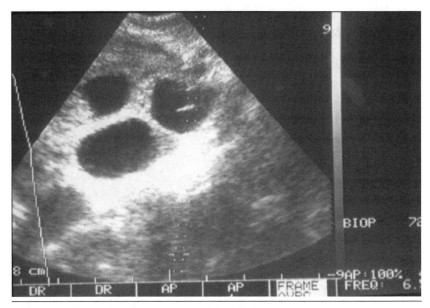

Figure 4.6. Multiple follicles during gonadotrophin therapy

(cytologists or embryologists) then IUI is the cheapest option although the pregnancy rate (19%) is not as high as intracytoplasmic sperm injection (ICSI; 26%). With the appropriate staff and facilities then IUI can be undertaken in the outpatients clinic of a general hospital. All other treatments for male infertility should be undertaken in specialist centres. ICSI is suitable for severe oligospermia and can sometimes be successful following testicular or epidydimal biopsy.

Men with Kleinfelter's syndrome or azoospermia should be referred to a specialist centre for consideration of donor insemination.

**Tubal disease.** Tubal surgery is still available in a few specialist centres but for the majority of women *in-vitro* fertilization offers the best chance of success.

**Psychological support.** Subfertility may be associated with significant levels of stress. The stress may be confined to one or other of the couple but often involves both of them. Considerable pressure is put on relationships particularly when the diagnosis is made and one of the couple is found to have a problem whilst the other does not.

The treatment can lead to sexual dysfunction or unmask an underlying problem such as erectile dysfunction. Couples therefore often need psychological support and it is helpful to be able to refer to a counsellor who has a particular interest in subfertility and/or is a qualified psychosexual counsellor. All assisted conception units have a counsellor as part of the requirements of the HFEA.

# Recurrent miscarriage

## Definition

Recurrent miscarriage (RM) is defined as the spontaneous loss of three or more pregnancies before the 24th completed week of pregnancy.

## Prevalence

RM is rare, affecting around 1% of couples. It is a very distressing condition often leading to serious psychological morbidity. Couples may separate because of the distress and desperation of their situation, the woman often starts to feel very ambivalent about being pregnant because of the psychological pain engendered by so many losses. Clinical depression is not uncommon and symptoms should be asked for. Fortunately 65% of couples will successfully achieve a live birth spontaneously and it is worth emphasizing this fact.

Since miscarriage may occur early (before 12 weeks gestation) and late (between 12 and 24 weeks gestation) in pregnancy there are different underlying causes. Occasionally a cause of RM can be found, more commonly conditions associated with miscarriage may be found in the mother and in many cases no cause or association is found. The amount of research into the condition is limited by our inability to do basic scientific experiments on the embryonic – maternal interface *in vivo* because of the risks to the developing embryo. Investigations are performed on the parents whilst the woman is not pregnant and therefore the ability to identify treatable causes is limited.

## Aetiology of RM

### Genetic

Abnormalities in the parental karyotype occur in 3–5% of couples. The most common abnormalities are balanced reciprocal translocations and Robertsonian translocations. Whilst these couples do have a reasonable chance of a sponta-neous successful pregnancy (40%) many couples find the strain of recurrent bereavement too much to bear and stop trying for a pregnancy. However, the development of pre-implantation genetic diagnosis (PGD) allows the couple to go through IVF, the embryos to be tested and only the normal embryos are replaced. IVF techniques do not have a high success rate in themselves (around 20% take home baby rate) and this is a limitation.

There is now evidence that embryos of couples with RM have a higher inci-dence of chromosomal abnormality than age matched controls. Studies in men from RM couples have shown an increased rate of chromosomal abnormalities in the sperm despite a normal peripheral karyotype. Currently this is at the research level only but may provide future treatment opportunities through PGD.

## PCOS

Polycystic ovaries are found in around 40% of women with RM. The underlying endocrine abnormality that predisposes these women to miscarriage has not been identified. Initially the raised LH concentration commonly found in women with PCOS was thought to be the primary factor associated with an increased risk of miscarriage. It is now thought that the raised LH may be a marker for another hormonal abnormality or an influence on the development of the ova or endometrium. Down-regulation of the pituitary with gonadotrophin releasing agonists has not been shown to improve the outcome of pregnancy.

PCOS has also been implicated in the concept of luteal phase defects. There is no correlation between serum progesterone levels and outcome of pregnancy and despite many studies, there is no evidence that progesterone support in early pregnancy improves the outcome of pregnancy.

### Hyperprolactinaemia

In one series around 18% of women with RM had raised prolactin levels. In a prospective randomized trial treatment resulted in a significantly better live birth rate than no treatment.

### Antiphospholipid syndrome

This syndrome is now the most important treatable cause of RM. Its diagnosis is a combination of clinical history (*Box 4.7*) and specific investigations looking for antibodies against the phospholipid binding proteins (anticardiolipin antibodies) and lupus anticoagulant.

The presence of both anticardiolipin antibodies and lupus anticoagulant on two occasions more than 6 weeks apart together confirm the diagnosis of antiphospholipid syndrome. The outcome of pregnancy in women who are left untreated is low with a live birth rate of around 10%. Randomized trials have shown that this can be improved to 40% if treated with low dose aspirin (75 mg daily) and improved still further with low molecular weight heparin

| Box 4.7 | Clinical obstetric criteria for the diagnosis of antiphospholipid syndrome |
|---|---|
| | 1. One or more unexplained deaths of a morphologically normal fetus at or beyond the 10th week of gestation, with normal fetal morphology documented by ultrasound or by direct examination of the fetus |
| | *OR* |
| | 2. One or more premature births of a morphologically normal neonate at or before the 34th week of gestation because of severe pre-eclampsia, or severe placental insufficiency |
| | *OR* |
| | 3. Three or more consecutive spontaneous miscarriages before the 10th week of pregnancy with maternal anatomic or hormonal abnormalities and maternal and paternal chromosomal causes excluded. |

therapy at thromboprophylactic doses. In women with only one or other of the APS tests proving positive the best treatment is with low dose aspirin alone since heparin does have a theoretical risk to the woman of developing osteopenia.

Women with APS are still at high risk of developing pre-eclampsia and the fetus is more likely to develop intrauterine growth restriction or deliver prematurely. This group should therefore be looked after in tertiary referral centres.

## Thrombophilic disorders

Thrombophilic defects such as mutations in Factor V Leiden or antithrombin III are associated with an increased risk of stillbirth, pre-eclampsia, abruption and intrauterine growth restriction. Unlike APS the effects of these abnormalities seem to affect the fetus in the second and third trimester of pregnancy. Seventeen percent of women with a thrombophilia have normal pregnancies so the precise risk cannot be identified. However, in women with recurrent second trimester loss, particularly with intrauterine death the presence of a thrombophilia should be investigated. As yet there is no evidence whether aspirin or heparin or both should be given to these women.

## Anatomical abnormalities

Congenital uterine anomalies have been named as a cause of RM and yet many women with uterine anomalies do have normal pregnancies. There is an association between premature delivery and a significant septum in the uterus but usually subsequent pregnancies deliver at later gestations thereby reducing the risks to the fetus and making surgical correction unnecessary. In women with a uterine anomaly and recurrent first trimester loss it is very unlikely to be due to the uterine anomaly. In recurrent late second trimester losses consideration of surgery should be undertaken very cautiously since there is a significant risk of subfertility from intrauterine scarring.

Cervical incompetence is a rare cause of RM and is usually secondary to therapeutic abortions performed on an unprepared cervix. The damage to the internal os usually occurs with forced dilatation beyond 10 mm. It can therefore follow both early and late surgical termination. A rare cause these days is following treatment for cervical abnormalities since the large loop excision technique very rarely damages the internal os. The history usually includes spontaneous rupture of membranes between 14 and 22 weeks with no prior pain. The baby may or may not have delivered spontaneously since once the membranes rupture the cervix often closes again and does not allow the baby to deliver. Its diagnosis can sometimes be made at HSG when the cervix balloons open as the dye is introduced or early in pregnancy by transvaginal scanning of the cervix. If the cervical length shortens or funneling is seen then a cervical suture should be inserted. If this fails then an interval cervical suture can be placed at the internal os.

Unexplained RM

In a large number of couples the investigations will not find an obvious abnormality that may be associated with miscarriage. This is often difficult for couples and a careful explanation that these investigations are only detecting a few conditions associated with RM that may exist in the parents. We are unable to do any research on the feto-maternal interface on a woman whilst she is pregnant. The outcome for future pregnancies in women under the age of 38 of normal BMI is

| Box 4.8 | Investigations for RM | |
|---|---|---|
| **All/1st trimester loss** | | |
| Parental peripheral blood karyotyping | Translocations | |
| | | |
| LH, FSH | | |
| PRL | PCOS, hyperprolactinaemia | |
| Testosterone | | |
| | | |
| USS | PCOS, uterine anomaly | |
| | | |
| Lupus anticoagulant | | |
| anticardiolipin antibodies (twice at least 6 weeks apart) | Antiphospholipid syndrome | |
| **2nd trimester loss** | | |
| HSG/HyCoSy | Uterine anomaly if USS abnormal | |
| | Cervical incompetence | |
| Thrombophilia screen | Factor V Leiden mutation, antithrombin III | |

| Box 4.9 | Treatment for RM | |
|---|---|---|
| **Diagnosis** | **Treatment** | |
| Unexplained | Supportive treatment | |
| PCOS (regular cycle) | | |
| | | |
| PCOS (oligomenorrhoea) | 1. Supportive treatment alone (if further loss –) | |
| | 2. Progesterone/hCG therapy to 14 weeks | |
| | | |
| Uterine anomaly | Supportive therapy ?? surgery | |
| | | |
| Cervical incompetence | Transvaginal scanning in pregnancy | |
| | Cervical cerclage per vagina | |
| | Cervical cerclage per abdomen | |
| | | |
| Antiphospholipid syndrome | | |
| Lupus anticoagulant alone (LA) × 2 | Aspirin 75 mg (pre pregnancy to 36 weeks) | |
| Anticardiolipin antibodies alone (ACA) × 2 | Aspirin 75 mg (pre pregnancy to 36 weeks) | |
| LA and ACA positive | Aspirin 75 mg + LMW Heparin to 36 weeks | |

on the whole good in these circumstances with a 65% spontaneous remission rate with no further intervention. This can be improved still further with reassurance or supportive care alone to 75%.

## Investigations

The investigations for all couples that have suffered with recurrent miscarriage are shown in *Box 4.8*. It is extremely rare for additional tests to be required and these should be applicable to the individual rather than applied across the board.

## Treatment

There have been many treatments advocated for RM. The majority have never been proven in randomized controlled trials. A summary of treatments that have been subject to randomized trials is shown in *Box 4.9*. No other treatments are recommended routinely.

# 5 | Oncology

## Introduction

The introduction of a 2-week maximum waiting time for patients who may have a malignancy means that the referral and appointment system must work efficiently and effectively. Chapter 1 deals with the handling of the referrals and appointments and the setting up of a rapid access clinic. This chapter will deal with the path that the patient follows through the rapid access clinic, completion of all investigations to admission if required.

## Ovarian cysts and pelvic masses

Referral letters that mention pelvic masses in women over the age of 50 should rouse suspicion of an ovarian malignancy, although large masses may also be found in younger women. Most GPs will arrange ultrasound scans prior to making the referral but if not already performed, an ultrasound scan of the pelvis and abdomen, CA125, CEA and CA199 should be requested by the senior doctor handling the referrals. The consultant's secretary should send the appropriate request forms directly to the patient. All patients should be seen in the clinic within 2 weeks from the date the referral letter is received.

If a scan has already been performed, then a copy of the results should be obtained and filed in the patient's notes. The management of the findings is outlined below and in *Figure 5.1*.

### The younger woman

Suitable for conservative management and rescan in 3 months (low risk for malignancy)

- pre-menopausal;
- unilocular, nonechogenic ovarian cyst of less than 5 cm in maximal diameter;
- no free fluid in the Pouch of Douglas;
- CA125 level less than 25.

If the patient is less than 30 years old, then a germ cell tumour must be suspected and serum AFP, Beta HCG, and LDH must also be requested along with CA125. If these are normal then the patient can be managed conservatively.

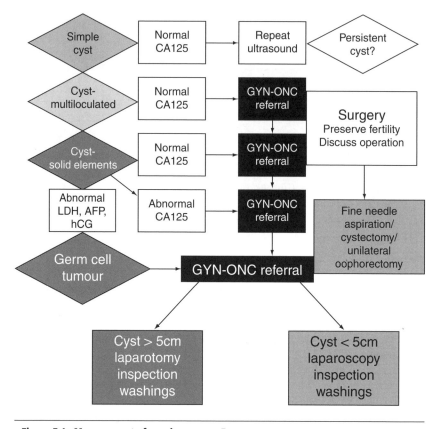

**Figure 5.1. Management of ovarian cysts > 5 cm**

Requires minimal surgical intervention

- pre-menopausal;
- unilocular nonechogenic cyst of over 5 cm;
- normal CA125 (less than 25).

Admit as day case for laparoscopy, peritoneal lavage and aspiration of ovarian cyst or ovarian cystectomy.

Suitable for simple ovarian cystectomy

- unilocular/multilocular ovarian cyst > 5 cm in maximum diameter with or without echogenic foci (dermoid cyst/cystadenomas);
- normal CA125 and other markers;
- age less than 40/wishes to preserve fertility.

Unilateral oophorectomy, omental biopsy and biopsy of the contra-lateral ovary

- multilocular, solid and cystic elements;
- presence of ascitic fluid;
- less than 35 years old;
- family not complete;
- raised βhCG/AFP/LDH levels;
- raised CA125.

Total abdominal hysterectomy, bilateral salpingoophorectomy (TAH + BSO) and omentectomy

- multilocular, solid and cystic elements;
- presence of ascitic fluid;
- raised CA125;
- over 35 years old;
- family completed.

### Women over the age of 45/post menopausal

Conservative management in this case should be reserved for those women who do not wish to have surgery and have negative ovarian tumour markers. If surgery is not performed then very careful follow-up is required with repeat scans and tumour markers every 3 months. If the cyst increases in size or morphology then unilateral oophorectomy with omental biopsy and peritoneal washings is the minimum intervention recommended. Ideally post menopausal women who develop ovarian cysts should have a TAH + BSO and omentectomy with peritoneal washings.

All patients who are suspected of having an ovarian cancer should be referred to a specialist gynaecological oncologist for full staging that includes sampling of para-aortic nodes.

## Post menopausal bleeding

Prior to the appointment it is essential that the woman has a trans-vaginal ultrasound scan to measure the endometrial thickness and assess the uterus and ovaries. This should be performed urgently if the GP has not arranged it or the patient should be given an ultrasound appointment on the day of her outpatient/rapid access appointment. The management of PMB is shown in *Figure 5.2*.

The results of the ultrasound scan should be in the patient's notes at the time of consultation. All women with PMB should have a speculum, cervical smear and bimanual examination.

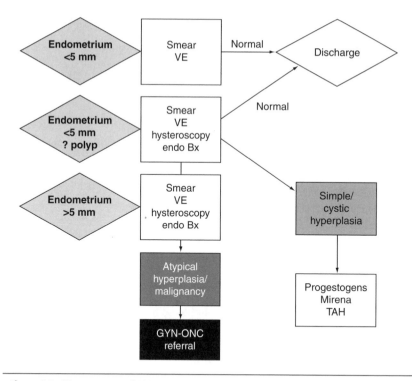

**Figure 5.2. Management of PMB**

## Endometrial thickness of less than 5 mm (8 mm if on HRT) and no other abnormality

Hysteroscopy is not required if this is the first episode of PMB. Speculum and vaginal examination must be performed in all cases to exclude cervical and vaginal lesions, and where these are present a punch biopsy must be obtained and sent for urgent histology. A cervical smear should also be obtained. If all these are negative, the patient may be reassured and discharged to the GP's care. The GP should be informed in writing and asked to refer the patient back to the clinic if PMB recurs. Oestrogen cream can be given vaginally for 10 days in these situations if atrophic changes are diagnosed in the genital tract.

### Endometrial thickness measures 5 mm or more

Hysteroscopy and endometrial biopsy should be performed at the clinic as part of the first appointment. All tissue obtained should be sent for **urgent** histology. A senior member of the medical staff should check all histology reports.

A register of all endometrial biopsy samples sent should be recorded in the clinic and all results from the previous week must be reviewed at the beginning of each clinic.

Where there is evidence of malignancy the patient should be referred urgently to the gynaecological oncologist. The pre-op work up should include full blood count, urea and electrolytes, liver function tests, chest X-ray and ECG.

If the histology shows endometrial hyperplasia or cellular atypia, the patient should be seen in the outpatients within 2 weeks to discuss treatment. In simple cystic hyperplasia then 6 months treatment with high dose progestogen or a Mirena IUS and a repeat endometrial biopsy is acceptable. If cellular atypia is present then a TAH with or without oophorectomy should be recommended.

If the histology is negative or benign, the patient and her GP should be notified and the patient discharged to the care of her GP. If examination and hysteroscopy show normal findings and no curettings are obtained then the patient is reassured and discharged back to her GP. Otherwise a follow-up appointment is arranged. The GP is asked to refer the patient back if the problem recurs.

# Management of cervical abnormality

The management of cervical disease requires coordination and agreement between primary care, general practitioners, cyto-pathology, gynaecological oncology, genito-urinary medicine and colposcopy.

## Post-coital bleeding

- PCB is **not** a symptom of pre-invasive cervical intra-epithelial neoplasia but can be a symptom of cervical cancer.
- PCB can be a symptom of several benign conditions including cervical polyps, cervical ectropion, cervicitis and coital trauma.
- PCB in women under the age of 25 is likely to be due to a benign cause rather than to cervical cancer. Those in this age group who are sexually active should be screened for chlamydia trachomatis infection, even if the examination shows no overt cervicitis and /or infection a referral to a genitourinary medicine clinic is indicated.
- When a patient presents with PCB, relevant history should be taken to verify the symptom. Examination of the cervix is mandatory to exclude visible signs of cancer, such as tumour or ulcer, or to make a diagnosis of cervical polyps, or overt cervicitis.
- If the most likely cause for PCB is felt to be primary cervical pathology then the patient should be referred to the rapid access clinic as an urgent referral, rather than via the colposcopy clinic.

### Persistent IMB, vaginal discharge

- If either the history or examination suggests cervical or other genital tract infection, then appropriate tests including chlamydia and/or referral to a genito-urinary medicine clinic are indicated. Women under 25 are a special risk group. It is essential that robust arrangements be made for following the patient up within a maximum of 2 weeks to ensure that further action to deal with the cause of PCB is being pursued.
- Young women who are on the OCP, progestogen only pill or long acting progestogens should only be given the diagnosis of breakthrough bleeding when all swabs and a cervical smear are negative.
- Examination of the cervix is mandatory to exclude visible signs of cancer, such as tumour or ulcer, or to make a diagnosis of cervical polyps, or overt cervicitis.
- If the most likely cause for IMB or vaginal discharge is felt to be primary cervical pathology then the patient should be referred to the rapid access clinic as an urgent referral, rather than via the colposcopy clinic.

Treatment of cervical disease depends on its cause. Infections should be treated appropriately and followed up with contact tracing via the genito-urinary medicine clinic. Cervical ectropion, abnormal smears should be treated in colposcopy or the minor procedures clinic with cryocautery or loop excision as appropriate. Cervical polyps can be removed in the clinic. An ultrasound scan and/or a hysteroscopy should be performed to exclude endometrial pathology (*Figure 5.3*).

## Management of vulval abnormalities

Vulval disease most commonly affects older women. This group of women are very reluctant to present to their GP because they find it embarrassing. Unfortunately this may mean that women present late with fungating vulval tumours. However, there are benign causes of vulval symptoms that are readily treated.

The commonest early symptoms of vulval disease are itching and dryness. These are most commonly due to benign conditions, which include:

- lichen sclerosus;
- vulval dystrophy;
- vulval intraepithelial neoplasia;
- oestrogen deficiency;
- vulval cancer.

Younger women may present with acute or chronic vulval pain. This may be due to:

- herpes simplex (often recurrent);
- vulvodynia.

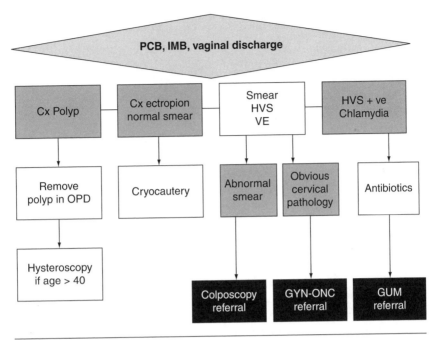

**Figure 5.3. Management of cervical pathology**

In lichen sclerosus or vulval dystrophy the vulva will have an area, or many areas, where the skin is whitened, smooth and thickened or thinned. Women with these conditions should be followed annually to detect early malignant change. The area may be bleeding because of being scratched excessively. It is important to biopsy these areas as there is a small risk of pre-malignant change. The biopsy can be performed under local anaesthetic in the minor procedures clinic.

If the woman is symptomatic and the vulva appears normal then it is worth doing a vulvoscopy to detect vulval intraepithelial neoplasia, which is graded similarly to cervical intraepithelial neoplasia. If this is positive then the vagina and cervix should be examined with the colposcope since all three are associated with human papilloma virus that in turn increases the risk of future malignant change.

If the skin is very thinned, the introitus very narrowed or the vulva fused in the midline then oestrogen deficiency is the obvious cause which can be resolved with oestrogen cream.

Areas that become ulcerated, have raised edges or bleed on contact are more likely to be malignant and a biopsy should be arranged urgently, preferably in the rapid access clinic. It is essential to examine the inguinal lymph nodes as this alters the prognosis.

Women with *de novo* herpes simplex may present with severe pain that in a few cases may cause urinary retention. Vesicles should be visible on examination. A rapid diagnosis from swabs and scrapes from the vesicles in the virology laboratory using PCR should be rapidly available. Recurrent cases tend to cause pain without obvious vesicles but there may be visible areas of inflammation on the labia.

Vulvodynia is a diagnosis of exclusion but classically touching two points at the introitus causes the pain and is diagnostic. Referral to a specialist vulval clinic is advised.

## Treatment

Steroid cream is the best treatment for vulval dystrophy, lichen sclerosus and vulvodynia. Some women with vulvodynia respond well to counselling in addition to medical treatment.

Oestrogen cream is usually beneficial for atrophic vulvitis. Sometimes surgery is required if the labia are fused together but this is rare.

Herpes simplex should be treated with acyclovir within 72 hours of development if its course is to be shortened. If the patient presents later than this then symptom relief is the best course of action whilst waiting for it to run its natural course.

Cases of vulval cancer should be referred to the oncologist for wide resection and lymph node biopsy.

# Colposcopy clinic

The size and set up of the colposcopy clinic will depend on the need in the catchment area. Clinics can either be held within the general gynaecology outpatient service or be in a dedicated area. Ideally this area should be within gynaecology outpatients or closely associated with it. The number of personnel and resources will vary depending on the number of referrals to the unit but the underlying principles will remain the same.

Colposcopy (diagnosis, treatment and surveillance) forms an essential part of the NHSCSP (National Health Service Cervical Screening Programme). As such it should be subject to the same or similar quality assurance measures as the laboratories performing cytology screening. The aim of the service should be to provide rapid access to accurate diagnosis and treatment for women who have an abnormality found in their cervical smear test. In addition the clinic should minimize intervention in women who do not have cervical intra-epithelial neoplasia.

## Staffing requirements

The service should have a designated lead clinician and lead nurse. There should be adequate numbers of qualified staff to ensure that all patients can be seen within the national guidelines for referral to appointment time (*Table 5.1*).

All colposcopists must be trained according to the British Society for Colposcopy and Cervical Pathology/Royal College of Obstetricians and Gynaecologists (BSCCP/RCOG) training programme.

Three roles are recognized for nurses within the colposcopy service:

- A designated nurse with specialist skills to assist in the running of the clinic. This nurse should not be seconded to other duties whilst the clinic is running. These nurses should be trained in the operation and sterilization of all the equipment used in the clinic.
- Nurses trained to perform colposcopy but not trained to perform treatment.
- Nurses trained in diagnostic and therapeutic colposcopy.

**Table 5.1.** Management of an abnormal smear result

| Smear result/condition | Action taken | Colposcopy appointment |
|---|---|---|
| Moderate to severe dyskaryosis | Immediate referral | Within 4 weeks |
| Mild dyskaryosis and borderline changes | The smear should be repeated in 3–6 months | Referral to colposcopy on the second occurrence of mild dyskarioysis and the third of borderline change |
| Suggestion of glandular neoplasia | Immediate referral | Within 4 weeks |
| PCB and abnormal looking cervix | | If there is a negative smear an appointment within 12 weeks. If there is any history of previous abnormal smears the appointment should be within 8 weeks |
| Any patient with an abnormal smear within 5 years of previous treatment | Referral to colposcopy | |
| Smear suggestive of invasive cancer | Immediate referral | Within 2 weeks |

Nurse specialists trained in colposcopy can deliver a highly effective and user sensitive service. Nurses should work with a lead clinician in a dedicated service. As with other providers in the service they should work to agreed guidelines and maintain their skills appropriately. It is the responsibility of the employing authority or Trust to ensure that nurse specialists in this field are given adequate opportunities to maintain their skill and knowledge base through attendance at national meetings and courses deemed appropriate by the lead clinician for colposcopy services.

The training for nurse colposcopists has been defined and is as for medical graduates. The only difference is that nurse training involves greater exposure to histopathology and cytopathology training in recognition that these components may not have been covered in as much detail in the basic training phase. As with medical trainees, the training programme should be the subject of continued review by the Joint Training Committee of the BSCCP.

## Referrals

Referrals to the clinic should be made in line with national guidelines but exceptions to this should be discussed with the lead clinician. The national guidelines are shown in *Table 5.1*.

Along with the standard clinic appointment letter all women should receive an information leaflet prior to their visit (*Box 5.1*). All women who are referred with an abnormal smear should be informed that they will have a colposcopic assessment prior to any treatment.

## Clinic environment

As with all gynaecology clinics there should be access to toilet facilities and each of the rooms should have a dedicated private area for changing. The rooms themselves should be set up as a consulting area with a computer terminal for results systems and EPR if in use. The computer database should be set up so that it can readily acquire and produce the annual returns that are now required by law as a quality assurance tool for the cervical screening programme (KC65). There should be a suitable couch, which can vary in height and a colposcope. There should be easy access to the equipment required for colposcopy and for treatment of CIN such as diathermy and cryocautery.

As in all clinic situations where procedures are carried out there should be access to resuscitation equipment and the staff should be fully trained in using this.

Equipment required:

- procedures couch;
- examination chair;
- light source;

Box 5.1 | Patient information

# AN ABNORMAL CERVICAL SMEAR

## *YOUR QUESTIONS ANSWERED*

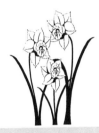

### An Abnormal (or Positive) smear result

What does it mean? An abnormal (or positive) smear result means that changes have occurred in the sample of cells that were taken from your cervix (neck of the womb – see diagram below) during the smear test. Having a smear test enables changes to be found at an early stage when they can be easily treated. Medical names for these changes are Cervical Intraepithelial Neoplasia (CIN), dyskaryosis and dysplasia. Some of these changes may in time develop into cancer. Therefore, it is important that you attend appointments for further investigation and treatment (if necessary). It is very rare for an abnormal smear to mean that you have cancer.

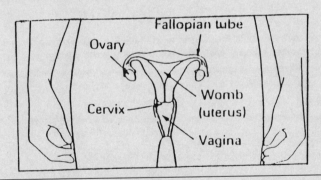

**Position of the cervix**

### Colposcopy examination

A Colposcope is a special microscope that enables the doctor to look closely at the cervix. This examination is done in the gynaecology outpatient department. Before the examination the doctor will ask you question about your medical history. You will then undress from the waist down (a skirt does not need to be removed) and be helped to get into a comfortable position on the couch. If a medical student wished to observe, your consent is obtained first.

A colposcopy **may not** be done your period. Please ring the clinic for further advice.

The vaginal walls are held open by an instrument called a speculum but no part of the colposcope goes inside you. A liquid is applied the cervix to highlight the abnormal area. One or two tiny samples of tissue (called biopsies) may be taken from the cervix. These are sent to a laboratory for a further check. Some women feel that the biopsy is painless while other find it hurts slightly. The colposcopy examination takes about 15–20 mins.

**Treatment *may either* be performed at the same time if necessary with your consent or we will write to you with the results. However, not everybody needs treatment. If this is the case you may be asked to have another smear test in 6 months as a further check.**

### Treatment

The most common treatment for women with CIN are *Loop diathermy* and *cold coagulation*. The *loop diathermy* uses a thin loop of electrified wire to remove the abnormal cells. This tissue is then sent to a laboratory to be examined. *Cold coagulation* involves destroying the abnormal cells by heat.

*Loop diathermy* and *cold coagulation* are very effective and do not damage the rest of the cervix. Both these treatments are carried out either in the Colposcopy Unit or the Day Surgery Unit. In the treatment room you will be helped to get on the couch and then given a local anaesthetic to prevent pain. A few women of however feel some period-like pain but this should not last very long.

*If you have a coil (IUCD), the doctor may take it out the time of your treatment. You should use an additional method of contraception (i.e. a condom) as well ad the coil or abstain from sex for 7 days before your appointment.*

In many respects these treatments are very like the colposcopy examination. You lie in the same position and the procedure takes about the same length of time (15 mins). If you feel shaky after the treatment you will be advised to sit down for a little while. *It is a good idea to bring someone along to take you home and to take things easy for the rest of the day. There is a small risk of heavy bleeding and/or infection after treatment. You will probably have light bleeding and discharge for up to two weeks or longer.*

**You should not have sexual intercourse or use tampons for a period of 4 weeks after treatment. It takes 4 weeks for the treated area to heal completely.**

The treatment is unlikely to affect fertility or the outcome of future pregnancy. The success rate of treatment is 90% – meaning one in ten women may need a second treatment.

### Cone Biopsy

A *cone biopsy* is recommended if all the abnormal area cannot be seen through the colposcope. This process both diagnoses the degree of abnormality and treats it at the same time. It involves the removal of a small cone-shaped piece of tissue from the cervix. It is done either by loop diathermy or by other surgical means, the tissue that is removed is examined in a laboratory to make sure it contains all the abnormal cells. The difference between a *cone biopsy* and the treatment described above is that a larger area of tissue is removed. Sometimes a general anaesthetic rather than a local anaesthetic is used. Occasionally a few days stay in hospital is required.

You should feel well after the treatment but are advised to take things easy for a week or so. It is important to avoid to much physical activity during this time because there is a slight risk of heavy bleeding. As with the other treatments, you will be told not to have sexual intercourse or use tampons for four weeks.

**If you have very heavy bleeding after any of the treatments you should contact your GP or come to the hospital casualty department at any time.**

### Follow-up appointment
You will be asked to attend for at least two further smears and/or colposcopy examination. The first six months after your treatment, followed by another six months later. This is to make sure that all the abnormal cells have been removed. It is therefore very important that you attend.

### Questions women ask about an abnormal smear result
*Have I got something seriously wrong?*
As mentioned above, it is very rare for an abnormal smear to mean that you have cancer, however, to prevent cancer from developing it is important that you attend all appointments.

*Will the treatment affect me having children?*
The treatments discussed above should not affect your ability to have children. Occasionally a cone biopsy will weaken the cervix. This may slightly increase the risk of miscarriage.

*Will treatment by successful?*
The above treatments have a very high success rate. Of over 90%. Occasionally it is necessary to repeat the treatment in order to remove all the abnormal cells.
*Will the abnormal cells get worse while I am waiting for my appointment?*
Changes usually take place of a long period of time. Therefore the abnormality should not get any worse while you are waiting for an appointment for colposcopy treatment.

*What causes abnormal cells?*
Unfortunately we cannot give you a precise answer to this question as no one knows the exact cause. There are several factors which may be linked to the development of CIN. These include:

**1.** Heavy smoking.

**2.** A common virus that may have been passed on during sexual intercourse.

**3.** The age at which a woman starts to have intercourse (the cervix of a teenager is more vulnerable to infection).

*Can I still have sexual intercourse?*
The abnormal cells themselves cannot be passed on to your partner. Therefore you can have a normal sexual life while waiting for a colposcopy examination or treatment. As mentioned above, after treatment you should not have sexual intercourse for 4 weeks.

Acknowledgement CANCER RESEARCH CAMPAIGN
REVISED: Dec 2001

- diathermy machine with patient pads;
- smoke extractor;
- colposcope;
- Matt cuscoes with extractor channel;
- decontamination and sterilization of instruments;
- cryocautery machine with three probes;
- disposable diathermy loop excisors in three sizes;
- disposable diathermy ball;

- diathermy leads and hand held diathermy delivery packs;
- silver nitrate sticks;
- iodine solution;
- acetic acid;
- sterile examination packs containing dental needle for cervical block;
- sterile gloves.

## Diagnosis and treatment

If cytology and colposcopy indicate high-grade disease (moderate to severe dyskaryosis, acetowhite grade 2–3) an outpatient loop excision of the transformation zone should be performed (LETZ). If there is CIN in the ectocervix and the transformation zone is not completely visible then a loop cone is indicated. If the ectocervix is normal and the patient is under 40 years old then an endocervical cytobrush can be performed with a 4-month follow-up. However, there are instances when a LETZ may need to be performed under a general anaesthetic. These are: wide excisions of lesions involving >90% of cervical area, the need for a knife cone (suspected invasive carcinoma), the patient's wishes or medical indications.

If the results are suggestive of low-grade abnormalities (borderline change or mild dyskaryosis with acetowhite grade 1) then the advantages and disadvantages of either surveillance or treatment can discussed with the patient according to the findings. If treatment is indicated/chosen then a LETZ or cold coagulation should be performed. Biopsies should be taken from the transformation zone prior to cold coagulation.

Surveillance can be carried out on women with low-grade abnormalities at the patient's request, this should be with 6-monthly smears and/or colposcopy.

## Treatment options

### Cold coagulation

This is effective for CIN but LETZ is preferable for high-grade disease. Prior to performing cold coagulation it has to be established that there is no suspicion of microinvasion, the transformation zone can be seen in its entirety and more than one punch biopsy is taken at the time of treatment.

The probe is applied to the abnormal area for 30 seconds at a temperature of 100–120°C. The conical ended probe should be used to ablate the transformation zone in the internal os.

### LETZ

This is a safe and effective treatment for CIN that can be performed in the outpatient clinic. It is the treatment of choice if the upper limit of the transformation zone is endocervical but visible and in women with high-grade disease. Loop cone biopsy should be considered if the upper end of the transformation zone is not visible, however, the patient will need to be warned of after effects and complications such as heavy bleeding, cervical stenosis and failure to treat completely. The main complication after this treatment is infection and the patient should be warned of how infection presents and who to contact if this arises.

A cervical block is given using xylocaine administered with a dental syringe to four points on the cervix. The loop is heated by diathermy and in a single bite a central core of the cervix is removed including the whole of the transformation zone.

### Knife cone biopsy

This should be performed under a general anaesthetic in a day surgery unit or main theatres if there is high-grade disease and the upper limits of the transformation zone are not visible at colposcopy. Another indication is microinvasive disease or for residual or recurrent disease after outpatient treatment.

### Hysterectomy

This is indicated in the presence of high-grade disease. If this is suspected then biopsies should be performed and the patient referred to the gynaecological oncologist.

## IUCD

Women may have treatment with the cold coagulator with their IUCD *in situ*. This needs to be removed for loop diathermy and the risk of pregnancy should be assessed and treatment rescheduled. The IUCD can be safely reinserted 6 weeks after treatment.

## Pregnant patients

Women can be seen from 8 to 30 weeks pregnant. A smear should be taken unless it has been performed in the last 3 months. Biopsies can be taken to exclude microinvasion. Treatment can be given if there is a suspicion of microinvasive or invasive disease.

## Menopausal patients

These patients may be difficult to assess unless they are receiving HRT. If the smear is high grade and the transformation zone is not visible a loop cone or knife cone is indicated particularly if the smear reports moderate to severe dyskariosis. In women with borderline smears and an incomplete colposcopy topical oestrogen may be indicated for 10 weeks prior to the colposcopy visit.

## Suspected invasion

The gynaecological oncologist should see women with smears suggestive of invasion within 2 weeks.

## Follow-up

A suggested regimen for follow-up is shown in *Table 5.2*.

**Table 5.2. Follow-up regimen**

| Biopsy result/treatment | Colposcopy appointment | Action required |
| --- | --- | --- |
| CIN 1 and opting for surveillance. | 6 months | Can be continued up to 2 years |
| If biopsy confirms CIN | A date for treatment should be given within 12 weeks | If this is to be performed in DSU then a form should be completed either within clinic or on receipt of the histology and the patient should discuss their date for the procedure with the admissions officers. |
| **Following cold coagulation:** | | |
| If the biopsies confirm CIN 1 | Discharge | 6 month follow up smear. |
| Higher grade | 6 monthly follow up | Smears by GP |
| **Following LETZ** | | |
| Resections of margins clear of CIN. | Discharge | GP for 6-month cytology follow up with spatula and brush |
| Resections of margins not clear of CIN. | 6 monthly follow up. | In colposcopy |

# 6 | Pelvic Floor Disorders

## Uterovaginal prolapse

Women are often referred to the gynaecology clinic with symptoms of uterovaginal prolapse, which are commonly associated with urinary problems. A prolapse can cause symptoms of:

- pelvic pain;
- local discomfort;
- ulceration and bleeding;
- backache;
- urinary and bowel symptoms.

The symptoms normally develop gradually. Prolapse may be secondary to medical disorders but is usually due to:

- inadequacy of the muscles or ligaments of the pelvic floor;
- obstetric factors;
- atrophy due to lack of oestrogen;
- an increase in intra-abdominal pressure.

There are four degrees of uterine prolapse:

- 1st degree – the cervix does not reach the introitus;
- 2nd degree – the cervix descends to the introitus;
- 3rd degree – the cervix is below the introitus;
- Procidentia – the uterus is outside the introitus.

However, there are types of vaginal prolapse that can occur independently of the uterus or after a hysterectomy:

- vault prolapse;
- cystocoele – the bladder bulges through the anterior vaginal wall;
- cysto-urethrocoele – this involves the urethra as well;
- enterocoele – a weakness in the upper third of the posterior vaginal wall;
- rectocoele – this is a prolapse in the middle third of the posterior wall, which lies adjacent to the rectum.

The treatment of a prolapse depends on the severity of the symptoms and the patient's wishes. These are normally surgical or conservative with the use of ring pessaries.

# Conservative therapy

Ring pessaries

**Indications for using a ring pessary.** Ring pessaries can be used instead of surgery in the management of uterovaginal prolapse. The main indications for use are:

- the patient does not want surgery;
- the patient is unfit for surgery;
- the patient's only symptoms are due to prolapse with minimal urinary symptoms;
- surgery carries a high risk of subsequent urinary problems.

Contraindications for use are:

- vaginal wall ulceration;
- recurrent urinary tract infections;
- 2nd or 3rd degree uterine prolapse;
- ulceration of the cervix;
- diabetes is a relative contraindication;

**Inserting/changing pessaries.** When undertaking this it is important to have all the equipment ready and in the consulting room.
  You will need to have:

- examination couch and light source;
- speculum;
- lubricating jelly;
- disposable gloves;
- warm water;
- selection of pessaries.

**The first visit.** A gynaecologist will usually insert the first ring pessary. The procedure is the same whether it is undertaken by a nurse or doctor. The patient should get undressed below the waist and be made as comfortable as possible on the couch. A full vaginal examination should be performed in the Sims position to establish the degree of prolapse and ensure that a ring pessary is the correct management. The health care professional should discuss and explain the procedure to the woman and obtain consent. The woman should be asked to go and empty her bladder. She should be asked to lie on her back.
  Selection of the correct ring size is made by measuring the length of the vaginal canal against the examiner's finger and then measured against the diameter of the ring pessary.
  The pessary should be able to rotate whilst *in situ* yet remain in place when the women is straining.

**Insertion of the pessary.** The most uncomfortable part of the procedure is the passage of the ring through the introitus. This is particularly true in women who have been post menopausal for many years. The pessary is very stiff and it helps to run the pessary under hot water for 5 minutes before insertion. Once it is more malleable the following should be done:

- Compress the pessary into an oval shape and apply lubricant onto the entering edge of the pessary.
- Part the labia and slide the pessary into the posterior part of the vagina.
- Continue gently sliding the ring backwards and downwards into the posterior fornix.
- The pessary should then spring into a circular shape.
- Insert a finger into the vagina and ensure that the distal part of the ring is in the posterior fornix so that the cervix is positioned centrally through the ring.
- Hook the front of the pessary into the anterior fornix so that it lies behind the symphysis pubis.
- Ask the women whether the pessary feels comfortable. She should walk round, cough, bear down and pass urine to ensure the pessary is correctly sited.
- She should be given contact telephone numbers if any problems arise prior to the next clinic visit.

**Subsequent visits.** The pessary should be changed every 6 months. At every visit an assessment of any symptoms must be made.

The symptoms to enquire about are:

- comfort of the pessary;
- presence or absence of prolapse symptoms;
- vaginal bleeding;
- vaginal discharge;
- sexual discomfort;
- urinary symptoms;
- problems defaecating.

If the patient has none of these symptoms nursing staff can change the pessary. For nurses to be able to undertake this they should have:

- an in-depth knowledge of the pelvic anatomy;
- be competent at passing a vaginal speculum and carrying out vaginal examinations;
- be able to recognize abnormal conditions of the vulva, cervix, vagina.

Ideally the nurse should have undertaken further educational courses in gynaecology or urogynaecology.

Removal of a pessary

- The vulva should be examined for lesions and signs of irritation prior to the removal of the pessary.
- To remove the pessary the labia are parted to expose the entrance to the vagina. One finger should be used to hook the proximal rim of the pessary where it lies in the anterior fornix behind the symphysis pubis. The ring should be pulled firmly but gently in a steady downward movement until the pessary comes out. This is usually quite uncomfortable and should be performed smoothly and quickly.
- A speculum should then be passed and the vagina examined for:
  (a) ulceration and excoriation caused by a poorly fitting pessary;
  (b) abnormal vaginal secretions and discharge, which may indicate an infection that needs to be treated prior to the replacement of the pessary
  (c) oestrogen deficiency, which will require topical oestrogen cream.
- If the examination is normal then the ring should be replaced as outlined above with the same size of ring.

If there are any substantial changes in the patient's symptoms then the nurse should contact the consultant gynaecologist and arrange for the patient to be reviewed.

## Surgery

The commonest operations for prolapse with minimal or absent bladder and bowel symptoms are a vaginal hysterectomy for uterine prolapse, anterior and/or posterior repair. These operations are effective in the short-term for improving symptoms but there is a high incidence of recurrence or a secondary prolapse occurring. This can be reduced by strong recommendations of a lifetime of pelvic floor exercises with support from nursing staff and/or physiotherapists. However, the first operation is the best chance of achieving long-term success.

New surgical procedures have been developed and ideally these women should be assessed and treated by specialists who have been trained in prolapse surgery. These new procedures include sacrospinous fixation and sacrocolpopexy.

# Incontinence and bladder dysfunction

As well as women presenting with a prolapse women will often arrive at the clinic with other problems related to their bladder.

## Definition of incontinence

The Department of Health has defined incontinence as 'the involuntary loss or inappropriate passing of urine and/or faeces that has an impact on social functioning or hygiene'.

It is a common experience amongst women with 10% of young women and 30% of women over the age of 60 turning to the health services for help with this embarrassing and important problem. Many more women suffer in silence.

Incontinence may take many forms.

### Stress incontinence

Stress incontinence is the involuntary loss of urine when intra-abdominal pressure increases during certain activities (i.e. coughing, laughing, standing, aerobics and sexual activities) and the bladder outlet is weak. This involuntary loss of urine occurs even though the bladder is stable/not contracting.

### Frequency

This is defined as passing urine more than eight times in a 24 hour period. This is a very common problem and may be related to some underlying bladder or gynaecology problem. It is most commonly associated with:

- UTI;
- during pregnancy;
- pressure from ovarian cysts and fibroids;
- local irritation;
- cystocoeles.

### Urge incontinence

The woman complains of a leakage of urine with urgent desire to void associated with frequency and nocturia. This is normally caused by detrusor instability and sensory urgency.

### Mixed urge and stress incontinence

The woman complains of symptoms of pure stress or urge incontinence or a mixture of both. This is normally due to incompetent sphincter and detrusor instability.

### Overflow incontinence

The patient complains of frequency, nocturia, passive dribbling, incomplete emptying of bladder and symptoms of a UTI.

### Voiding difficulties

The causes of voiding difficulties vary. Primary causes are often associated with medical conditions such as diabetes mellitus or multiple sclerosis. Secondary causes may be as a result of trauma or following surgery for incontinence or spinal problems. The patients most commonly present with retention or overflow incontinence.

Bladder problems and disorders all need to be assessed thoroughly by a competent health care professional. This is one area where there is increasing scope for the role of the nurse in the assessment and conservative treatment of women with pelvic floor disorders as the following sections will show.

The remainder of this chapter deals with stress incontinence, detrusor instability and voiding difficulties.

## Stress incontinence

Stress incontinence is by far the most common form of incontinence in women. It affects at least 40–50% of all women. Only a quarter of all women with the problem seek help.

### Definition

It is usually associated with:

- incompetent urethral sphincter;
- pregnancy and childbirth;
- obstetric trauma;
- laxity of the pelvic floor;
- prolapse;
- atrophy of the pelvic supports;
- oestrogen depletion;
- obesity;
- chronic constipation.

The main cause is because of weakness of the pelvic floor muscles. They are attached from the pubic bone in front and the coccyx behind. A strong, healthy pelvic floor muscle will help to support the internal organs, help to support the bladder and bowels, and also increase pleasure during sex.

### Aetiology of stress incontinence

Incontinence in women is due to an intrinsic loss of urethral strength. Childbirth and ageing weaken the urethral sphincter muscles. Childbirth also causes denervation of the nerve supply to the pelvic floor and sphincter muscle. The stretching of the pelvic floor during delivery will predispose to pelvic floor weakness. Other factors that worsen or predispose women to develop stress incontinence include obesity, chronic cough, and low oestrogen concentrations.

### Management of stress incontinence

Stress incontinence in women may be associated with detrusor instability. It is therefore important to identify this during the initial assessment to ensure that the condition is treated correctly.

A careful history should be taken which should include a description of the symptoms of stress incontinence (*Box 6.1*) as well as a full medical, surgical, obstetric and gynaecological history. Particular attention should be paid to a history of respiratory or neurological illnesses as well as chronic conditions such as asthma and diabetes. The number of cigarettes smoked per day is also important.

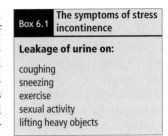

Examination of the patient should include the patients weight and height, blood pressure and examination of the respiratory system. A full neurological examination should be performed in patients with a history suggestive of a neuropathic bladder. A full assessment of the pelvic floor should be performed.

The examination should only be performed by a practitioner who is competent to do so.

- The patient should be examined in a supine position with her knees bent up and abducted laterally.
- The presence of any cystocoele (prolapse of the anterior vaginal wall) or rectocoele (prolapse of the posterior vaginal wall) should be noted. If either of these is severe, or if there is any degree of uterine descent, the chances of success from conservative management may be diminished.
- The presence of excoriation may give an indication of the severity of the incontinence.
- Examination of the introitus and distal vagina will identify the presence of vaginitis, where the vagina appears as a red, dry membrane instead of a moist, pink tissue. This is more common in post menopausal women and often mirrors the state of the urethra. Urethritis may cause frequency, urgency and dysuria.
- Ask the patient to cough. The assessor should observe for urinary leakage during the cough and record. There may also be demonstrable perineal descent, the vagina may bulge and gape and there may be movement of any prolapse
- The pelvic floor should be examined by inserting a gloved, lubricated finger into the vagina.
- Two fingers can be used to assess the strength, endurance and coordination of the pelvic floor
- The patient is asked to squeeze, lift, hold and relax. The examiner should feel the fingers being gripped and pulled inwards. Many women cannot do this at the first try, or tend to bear down or contract the abdominal muscles or buttocks.
- The strength of the muscle squeeze is noted using the Oxford Grading System (see below) as a guide. The length of time that the muscle is contracted is recorded in seconds. The woman must be in control of the

relaxation of the muscles so it should be noted at what point the contraction has faded away. It is futile to tell a woman to contract for 6 seconds when she is only able to contract for 4.

- It is then important to assess muscle endurance by getting the patient to contract, hold and release the muscle as many times as they can. This assesses the slow twitch muscles, which are responsible for the endurance and strength qualities.
- The 'quick twitch' movement of the muscle should then be assessed and recorded. This part of the exercise re-educates the part of the muscle responsible for the reflex activity. It should be noted how many can be done before fatigue sets in.
- The correct exercise programme should then be developed. The exercises may be worthwhile especially if the patient is keen and waiting for surgery. The exercises will improve the tone and blood supply locally thus improving postoperative healing.

The grade, strength and duration of muscle contraction can be assessed using the modified Oxford Grading System

The scale is as follows:

- 0 = nil
- 1 = flicker
- 2 = weak
- 3 = moderate
- 4 = good
- 5 = strong

### Initial treatment and baseline observations

- Send off urine sample to exclude a urinary tract infection.
- Ensure comprehensive assessment is completed.
- Complete frequency volume chart for 2 days recording input and output and any episodes of leakage.
- Refer to physiotherapist/continence nurse specialist for pelvic floor exercises.

### Conservative treatment

The following conservative therapies may be used to treat women with stress incontinence, but must only be used under the supervision of a competent practitioner. The patients must be followed up regularly, given encouragement and their progress monitored. It is possible to use a combination of the conservative measures, as pelvic floor exercises alone may not improve the symptoms:

- pelvic floor exercises;
- vaginal cones;

- intravaginal pessary;
- electrical stimulation;
- devices i.e. Neen pelvic floor educator, continence guards, perineometers, contiform;
- bladder training and general education;
- biofeedback.

**Pelvic floor exercises.** Strengthening of the pelvic floor muscles by regular exercise is the best form of therapy for mild to moderate stress incontinence, in absence of marked prolapse of the anterior vaginal wall. To achieve a successful outcome, it is imperative that the patient is well motivated and sufficiently mentally alert to carry out an exercise programme.

Exercising the pelvic floor muscles can strengthen them so that they provide good support. This will help to improve bladder control and improve or stop the leakage of urine. Like any other muscles in the body, the more they are used and exercised, the stronger they will become, so it is vital that patients are aware of how to do pelvic floor exercises correctly.

It is essential that the exercises are taught and performed correctly. Pelvic floor exercises are the most effective treatment for genuine stress incontinence provided the patients are taught correctly. They have been shown to be more effective than vaginal cones, or electrical stimulation or no treatment.

How to teach pelvic floor exercises

- Explain the reasons for pelvic floor weakness, i.e. childbirth, menopause, ageing.
- Explain the reasons for strengthening the pelvic floor muscles using diagrams/visual aids- this may help the patient to understand her condition better. It is important that everyday language should be used and medical terminology should be avoided if possible.
- Explain how to do pelvic floor exercises.
- Obtain consent and assess the pelvic floor (see p.116)
- Measure and record strength and hold using the Oxford Scale. This will enable you to assess progress made at future visits. It also gives the assessor an idea of the strength of the muscle before regular exercising. It provides you with a baseline reading/measurement.
- Measure the number of fast twitch exercises she is able to do before tiring.
- Set the exercise programme, explaining the importance of both the slow and fast twitch exercises in the strengthening of the pelvic floor muscle.
- Give out a leaflet explaining how to do pelvic floor exercises for the patient to refer to when she gets home.

- Give out information on hygiene, fluids to drink and avoid, the importance of preventing constipation, keeping weight steady etc.
- A Neen Pelvic Floor Educator can be given out at this stage if desired. They are useful if the women are unsure about the correct way to contract the pelvic floor muscles as they provide positive feedback when the correct muscles are used.
- Arrange follow-up treatment.

| Box 6.2 | How to use vaginal cones |
| --- | --- |

- Wash the cones and weights in soapy water and dry thoroughly.
- Hold the larger cone where it joins the cord and push gently into the vagina with only the cord remaining on the outside. When the cone is properly inserted in the vagina, the patient should be able to easily touch the bottom of the cone with her finger. It should not be inserted as high into the vagina as a tampon. If the cone is inserted too high into the vagina, it will make the exercises less effective.
- Keep the fingers on the point where the cord joins the cone and tighten the pelvic floor muscles. If the patient is contracting the correct muscles, then the cone should pull away from their finger. If the cone pushes onto their finger, then they are most probably pushing down with their stomach muscles.
- It is essential that this part of the procedure is taught correctly and that the teacher is happy that the patient is able to contract the pelvic floor muscle correctly as it will make a difference to the results achieved.
- Once the larger cone is inserted, stand up. Use the pelvic floor muscles to hold the empty cone in the vagina
    If this is not possible, then get the patient to lie down with the knees bent and the feet flat on the surface they are lying on. Tighten the pelvic floor muscles whilst gently pulling on the cord as if trying to pull it out. Tighten the pelvic floor muscles ten times, then stand up and try to hold the cone in place. If this is still not possible, then try again in the morning. It may be necessary to try some other pelvic floor stimulation if the muscles are very weak.
    If this is possible, then weights can be added to help strengthen the muscles.
- Unscrew the empty cone in the middle. Add the smallest weight to the spindle inside.
- Insert cone into the vagina.
- Walk around for 1 minute trying to retain the cone in the vagina, if the cone is held in place then increase the weight of the cone.
- The heaviest cone that can be actively retained for 1 minute by contracting the pelvic floor muscles is taken as a standardized measure of the pelvic floor muscle strength.
- The patient should then begin to exercise with the heaviest weight that she can still retain comfortably for 1 minute.
- She should aim to increase the time that she is able to retain the cone, up to a maximum of 15 minutes and to repeat this twice a day.
- Once she can hold the cone for a good 15 minutes, she can move up to the next heavier weight.
- Initially, the patient should concentrate on holding the cone in place, but once the muscles become stronger, she could increase the amount of movement by walking around.
- Since urinary incontinence occurs during stair climbing, running, coughing and hand washing, following an additional programme may be useful before moving up to a new weight.
    (a) Holding the cone while stair climbing, both up and down the stairs.
    (b) Holding the cone for 1 minute whilst running on the spot.
    (c) Holding the cone during 5–15 repeated coughs.
    (d) Holding the cone whilst hand washing for 1 minute.

Follow-up

- Follow-up within 6 weeks, 4 if possible.
- Reassess pelvic floor contraction.
- If contracting correctly and noticed an improvement, see in 4 months. Alter the exercise programme if necessary.
- If not contracting correctly, advise and see again in 6 weeks.
- Consider the use of vaginal cones and electrical stimulation.
- Refer to gynaecologist if unable to improve pelvic floor strength and hold or is still leaking. If considering surgery, then refer for urodynamic investigations.
- Discharge once able to contract the pelvic floor with good strength and hold, with no leaking.

**Vaginal cones.** Vaginal cones are plastic cones that are inserted into the vagina with varying weights inside. They help to strengthen the pelvic floor. When used correctly, cones provide a positive feedback of muscle progress, thus giving a sense of achievement. Pelvic floor muscle exercises with vaginal cones have been shown to be effective also in treatment of the symptoms of urgency that is often associated with the symptoms of genuine stress incontinence.

Since the use of cones requires very little professional time to teach, compared to conventional exercises, it represents a very cost effective option for the conservative management of stress incontinence (*Box 6.2*). There are some instances when vaginal cones are not advisable. Patients must be told about basic safety when using the cones (*Box 6.3*).

It is important to mention that due to the fatigue of the pelvic floor muscles during the day, many patients can retain heavier weights in the morning than in the evening.

Due to the variation in vaginal secretions, which affect cone retention, patients may demonstrate 'good' and 'bad' days. Pelvic floor muscles may appear weaker pre-menstrually.

**General advice.** Advice on the amount and type of fluids to drink in a 24-hour period is essential information to give all women attending the clinics. It is widely recommended that patients should drink eight cups (1.5 l/2.7 pints) of fluid a day to flush the bladder regularly to remove

| Box 6.3 | **When not to use vaginal cones** |
|---|---|

- When a moderate to severe vaginal prolapse is present
- When pregnant
- If a vaginal infection is present or suspected.
- During menstruation
- For 2 hours after sexual intercourse
- When muscle strength is below grade 3 on the Oxford grading scale.

**Safety issues**
- It is essential that the cones and weights are washed in between each use in soapy water and dried thoroughly. This will help to prevent infections such as thrush.
- Vaginal cones should never be shared between two people.

waste products and other irritants. It is common for people with bladder dysfunction to reduce their oral intake, which can in turn impact on already existing symptoms.

It is also important for women to have regular bowel movements as straining associated with constipation can cause pelvic floor muscle weakness. Advice on diet, position on the toilet and fibre intake can help to ease/solve any existing constipation problems.

Chronic chest problems associated with smoking may result in stress incontinence if the pelvic floor muscles are weak. Women should be advised to give up smoking and given the relevant literature and contact numbers for support in achieving this.

Symptoms may worsen if the woman develops a urinary tract infection. Advice should be given on hygiene, not using perfumed soaps, not wearing nylon underwear and drinking cranberry juice.

**Surgery.** If conservative therapy fails and the patient and doctor are considering surgery, then urodynamics must be performed to confirm diagnosis of genuine stress incontinence. Videourodynamics should be performed if the patient has a complicated history or has had previous surgery to the bladder.

Operations performed for women with genuine stress incontinence include:

- colposuspension;
- sling procedures i.e. tension-free vaginal tape (TVT);
- periurethral injectables i.e. collagen, macroplastique;
- anterior colporrhaphy;
- complex surgical procedures i.e. artificial sphincter.

## Management of detrusor instability

### Definition

Detrusor instability has been defined by the International Continence Society as 'the occurrence of uninitiated detrusor contractions that exert a pressure greater than 15 cm water during bladder filling while the patient is inhibiting the desire to void.

Detrusor contractions below 15 cm water may be clinically significant if associated with the symptoms of frequency, nocturia and urgency or micturition'.

The aetiology of detrusor instability may be:

- Idiopathic in which uninhibited detrusor contractions occur in a neurologically normal individual.
- Obstructive which is seen most commonly in association with bladder outlet obstruction (urethral stenosis in women).

- The result of detrusor hyper-reflexia in which uninitiated detrusor contractions occur in the presence of an underlying neuropathy, (i.e. MS, spinal cord injury.).

### Presentation

The symptoms associated with detrusor instability include:

- frequency;
- urgency;
- nocturia;
- urge incontinence;
- stress incontinence.

Patients must be asked specific questions about the frequency of micturition and the diurnal variation. They should be asked about fluid intake and medication that may be contributing to the problem.

### Baseline observations and investigations

- Send off urine sample for MC&S to exclude any urine infection. Treat accordingly if result comes back positive.
- Complete a baseline chart/frequency volume chart for 2 days recording input and output in millilitres and any episodes of leakage. If the chart shows irregular, small volume voids then it indicates detrusor storage dysfunction
- For a patient to be given the diagnosis of detrusor instability, they must have undergone urodynamic investigations. It is recommended that the patient is referred for urodynamics if conservative measures are unsuccessful or a definite diagnosis is required.

## Treatment of detrusor instability

### Medical treatment

The rationale for drug treatment in detrusor instability is to lessen detrusor over-activity by blocking parasympathetic transmission. Drugs with an anticholinergic action are generally effective (i.e. oxybutynin and tolterodine)

The patient should be warned of the possible common side effects of dry mouth, constipation, blurred vision. By lessening detrusor contractility, bladder emptying may be impaired and occasionally urinary retention can occur.

The patient should be given a leaflet with the titration guidelines for these medications. They should read it thoroughly with the doctor/nurse explaining any areas that needs to be clarified. The clinician should review the dose of tablets every 2 weeks and increase/decrease if necessary.

### Conservative measures

For the most effective results, patients suffering with urgency, frequency, nocturia and urge incontinence whose symptoms are affecting their quality of life should be referred to the continence advisor/nurse specialist. Bladder retraining, pelvic floor exercises and drug therapy should be used at the same time.

- **Bladder retraining** is an effective treatment for detrusor instability in motivated patients.
- Bladder training may be used alone or in conjunction with medication, the latter probably being more effective.
- **Changes in lifestyle** may lead to improvement in symptoms, i.e. looking at fluid intake and types of fluid drunk each day, eliminating stimulants such as caffeine from the diet.

### Bladder retraining

Bladder retraining programmes are most suitable for people with symptoms of **urgency, frequency and urge incontinence**, with or without an underlying unstable detrusor muscle, and for those with a non-specific incontinence, which they are unable to account for, and seem to 'just happen'.

Patients with a bladder dysfunction other than an unstable bladder are less likely to benefit from bladder training. (Symptoms of stress incontinence, or retention with overflow incontinence.) This highlights the need for a thorough assessment and accurate diagnosis prior to the implementation of any treatment programme.

The aim of bladder training is to restore the patient to a more normal and convenient micturition pattern and to give the individual confidence in their bladder's ability to hold onto urine. The objective is that voiding should occur only every 3–4 hours, or even longer without any urgency or urge incontinence.

When the bladder is known or thought to be unstable, drug therapy is often combined with bladder training (see management of detrusor instability)

*How to teach bladder training*
- The patient must be motivated.
- The patient should fill in a baseline chart/frequency volume chart for 48 hours in the week leading up to the appointment. This will give an idea of:
  (a) fluid intake;
  (b) frequency of micturition;
  (c) time in between each void;
  (d) frequency of leakage of urine;
  (e) volumes voided;
  (f) it will also provide a baseline for the patient to refer back to, to monitor their progress thereby aiding biofeedback.

- The clinician should provide information about normal bladder function including the knowledge that the bladder first signals an urge to empty when it is about half full.
- It should be explained that the bladder has become 'excited' or 'overactive' and so contracts when it shouldn't giving the urge to go to the toilet sometimes associated with urge incontinence.
- The patient should be advised to attempt the bladder training during the day only.
- The patient should be advised when she gets the urge to pass urine, to hold on and delay voiding for as long as she is able. This will allow the bladder to stretch and hold more urine.
- If the urgency is very strong they should be advised to sit and try to relax all muscles and deep breathe rather than rushing to the toilet when the first urge to empty the bladder is perceived.
- It may be necessary to advise the patient to hold on and delay voiding for a specific length of time, i.e. 15 minutes, and once that is achieved, to increase the time to half an hour, then 1 hour etc. For many women a 2–2.5 hour interval between voiding is more tolerable than a 3–4 hour interval.
- The patient must be given an instruction leaflet and another baseline chart to fill in for 24 hours in the week leading up to their next appointment.
- It is advisable to see the patients for their first follow-up appointment in approximately 4 weeks' time.
- They should also be given a pelvic floor exercises leaflet and asked to read it through. They should be taught how to perform pelvic floor exercises at a later consultation as there is a lot of information for one session and it is important that they retain as much information as possible. It is important that they learn how to contract their pelvic floor muscles so that when they get the urge to pass urine, they are able to tighten the muscles of the pelvic floor to help prevent leakage and enable them to hold on for longer.

*Practical advice for patients:*

- Patients must be warned that they may leak more at the beginning of the bladder-training schedule since the bladder is being stretched when it is holding onto larger volumes of urine.
- They must be warned that they will not notice changes immediately. Their bladder has taken time to get into the bad habit and will take time to get back into a good habit.
- They should regularly fill in the baseline chart to monitor their progress.
- They should be followed up regularly, every 4–6 weeks to start with, to maintain enthusiasm and motivation.
- They should be given lots of positive feedback when the baseline charts are compared and improvements are noted.

*General advice should include:*

- The patients should be advised to drink seven to eight cups of fluid a day.
- They should be advised on the effect of caffeine on their bladder, and advised to cut down the number of caffeinated drinks they consume.
- They should be advised on the importance of keeping their bowels regular and eating a healthy well balanced diet.

## Voiding difficulties

The causes of voiding difficulties vary. Primary causes are often associated with medical conditions such as diabetes mellitus or multiple sclerosis. Secondary causes may be as a result of trauma or following surgery for incontinence or spinal problems. The patients most commonly present with retention or overflow incontinence.

### Treatment

Medication may help in this condition. The commonest drug used is bethanocol, an alpha sympathomimetic that works by increasing the contractility of the detrusor muscle. The alternative is intermittent self-catheterization (ISC). Catheterization is invasive and should only be performed when all other possibilities have been explored and excluded. The patient requires individual assessment and the final decision to proceed should be made jointly with the patient, nurse and doctor.

ISC involves the patient inserting a catheter into the bladder via the urethra or cystostomy to drain off the urine. It needs to be taught in a sensitive way with maximum privacy.

Indications for ISC:

- retention, chronic and acute;
- hypotonic/atonic bladder;
- to measure residual urine;
- incontinence management for overflow as a last resort;
- neurological disease, neuropathic bladder- MS, stroke, paralysis;
- administration of intra-vesical medication;
- to obtain a sterile specimen of urine;
- incomplete bladder emptying;
- post urethrotomy for stricture therapy.

ISC should not be performed if a urethral device is already present, or if the patient gains sexual satisfaction from inserting the catheter . ISC is difficult to accept in some cultures and sensitivity is required when discussing it as an option. It is essential to obtain full consent and to have given the patient full written information before undertaking to teach ISC.

Teaching ISC

A qualified nurse who can demonstrate competence should teach ISC. The following equipment is needed to ensure aseptic technique:

- apron;
- gloves – sterile and non-sterile;
- sterile catheter pack;
- cleaning fluid e.g. Normasol;
- correct type of catheter;
- sterile water to soak the lubricated catheter;
- sterile jug if measurements are required;
- urinalysis stix;
- mirror.

*Procedure*
- Introduce oneself.
- Explain procedure and reasons for undertaking ISC.
- Check for allergies.
- Gain the patient's consent and document – verbal consent is usually adequate.
- Get patient to void into the measuring jug and measure amount passed.
- Wash hands.
- Put on apron.
- Clean trolley and set up sterile field with catheter pack, cleaning fluid and sterile gloves.
- Help patient into correct position on the couch. When first teaching ISC ensure that patient is sitting or is supine on couch. They must feel comfortable and safe.
- Set up mirror in position and demonstrate the meatus to the patient.
- Patient and nurse should put on sterile gloves
- Assist the patient to clean the meatus observing for vaginal discharge, urethral bleeding, meatal erosion and meatal sores.
- Prepare self-lubricating catheter by opening the funnel end 5 cm and filling with sterile water. Use adhesive tab to secure catheter whilst soaking.
- Leave catheter to soak for 30 seconds. Ensure manufacturer's guidelines are followed for the catheter being used.
- Assist the patient to insert the catheter into the bladder
- Allow urine to drain. Observe urine for clarity, odour, colour, and contents. Record volume of urine.

- Remove the catheter. Stop on removal if more urine drains. Remember the time factor because of the drying out effect of the catheter. Putting a finger over the end of the funnel until it is removed may help to prevent spillage.
- Assist patient to get dressed.
- Dispose of equipment into yellow bags.
- Wash hands.
- Perform urinalysis on the specimen. If it indicates a possible infection (leucocytes, blood and nitrites) then send off sample for culture.

The following details **must** be documented:

- date and time of catheterization;
- signature of nurse teaching the catheterization;
- state reason for catheterization and any problems encountered;
- brand of catheter used;
- material it is made of and its size (Ch);
- length;
- batch number;
- pre-void amount of urine passed and residual drained during catheterization;
- catheterization frequency and personal programme;
- follow-up dates.

It is advisable to have a data sheet to fill in for these patients and a facility for entering their details on an ISC database.

Before the patient leaves the department the nurse should do the following:

- give the patient an ISC booklet;
- give the patient a contact number and name;
- give advice on fluids including cranberry juice therapy;
- give advice on keeping bowel movement regular;
- give the patient some product information – where to get supplies, how to dispose of catheters, mail order home delivery service, nurse help-line;
- warn of the possible risks associated with ISC – Infections, inability to remove the catheter, pain, small amount of bleeding;
- give the patient details of follow-up, and an ISC programme.

Initially the patient should catheterize four times daily for the first fortnight. The patient should record the residual drained from the catheter in their ISC booklet which they should bring to each clinic appointment.

*Follow-up*
- Ring the patient the next day to check on their progression.
- See in 2 weeks for first follow-up unless the patient is contacted and they are having problems.

- Look at residual chart and reduce/increase the amount of catheterizations per day depending on the residual volumes.
- It is not advisable to treat UTIs if they are asymptomatic.
- The patients should be seen a minimum of 6-monthly and never discharged from nursing care whilst they are performing ISC.

## Urodynamic investigations

Urodynamics are invasive and embarrassing investigations and therefore only women who would benefit from this investigation should be referred.

Who requires urodynamics?

- Women who are likely to need bladder neck surgery.
- Women who have had bladder neck surgery and who still have significant urinary symptoms.
- Women who have failed simple conservative therapy for urinary symptoms.
- Women who have complex urinary symptoms or in whom you suspect a neuropathology.
- Women with prolapse who have or have had significant urinary symptoms and who are to undergo surgery.
- Women who have significant urinary symptoms the cause of which is unsure.

### Who requires uroflowmetry in clinic and a urinary residual?

- Patients who have irritative bladder symptoms, namely frequency (greater than eight voids per day) nocturia (greater than one void per night), urgency and urge incontinence who do not fulfil the criteria for urodynamic investigations.
- Patients who have symptoms of voiding difficulties, or recurrent urinary tract infections or haematuria. (The latter may also require cystoscopy and further investigations and should be discussed with the consultant.)

If women have uncomplicated stress incontinence or overactive bladder they should be managed initially with simple conservative therapy and referred to the continence nurse specialist. They may need to be prescribed anticholinergic therapy after a standard continence assessment.

## Equipment required for the investigation

The equipment required is shown in *Box 6.4* and *6.5*.

| Box 6.4 | Equipment needed for urodynamic test |
| --- | --- |

- Urine flow meter
- Infusion pump and giving set
- Urodynamic machine
- Infusion fluid – water for simple cystometry-urograffin for videourodynamics

## Staff and their training requirements

It is essential that urodynamic studies are carried out or supervised by experienced investigators. If videocystourethrography is being offered (which it should be for a complete service) then ensure that the investigator is competent at using the X-ray machine and has done the POPUMET course.

The investigator will have a full and in-depth knowledge and understanding of urinary incontinence and the possible treatment options

| Box 6.5 | Equipment needed for catheterization |
| --- | --- |

- Catheter pack
- 10Fr Nelaton filling catheter
- Instillagel
- Cleaning agent
- KY jelly
- Rectal line with hole in balloon
- Intravesical line
- Sterile gloves and apron

## Preparation for the clinic visit

The patient should have been sent a leaflet outlining the procedure with the appointment letter. The leaflet should include a contact number for the continence advisor or specialist nurse so that the patient can ring with any anxieties or questions. Enclosed with the appointment should be a quality of life questionnaire and a voiding chart. The instructions in the appointment letter should include the request for the patient to complete these and bring them with her.

## The clinic visit

On arrival the continence nurse should fully explain the test to the woman and check that the patient fully understands the procedure. She should also:

- collect quality of life questionnaire and clear up any misunderstandings or queries that it has created;
- look at voiding chart;
- ask women of childbearing age whether there is a chance that they could be pregnant and when their last period was. If the patient is unsure, then do a pregnancy test. Document all results;
- ask whether the patient has any allergies and record.

## The procedure

- Encourage the patient to void into the flow meter.
- Help up onto the couch after removing underwear.
- Explain the procedure and reassure throughout the test.
- Put on apron and gloves and clean perineal area and labia. (Clean from front to back.)
- Put on sterile gloves.
- Locate urethra and insert instillagel to lubricate and anaesthetize urethra.
- Wait 2–3 minutes to allow anaesthetic properties to work.
- Piggy back filling catheter and intravesical catheter and insert into the bladder. Ensure they are disengaged once in the correct position.
- Ensure rectal line has a hole in the balloon and insert into the rectum past the anal sphincter.
- Measure residual from bladder and dipstick. If positive to nitrites, leucocytes and blood discontinue test and commence on course of antibiotics.
- Attach filling catheter to giving set.
- Tape all three lines to the inner thigh to prevent them falling out.
- Attach rectal and intravesical lines to the transducers on the machine and flush with saline ensuring that all air bubbles and leaks have been removed. Failure to remove bubbles will lead to errors in measurement.
- Balance both lines to air.
- Get patient to cough to ensure that all lines are subtracting effectively and then at minute intervals throughout the test. This ensures that quality control is maintained.
- Start to fill bladder with sterile water at 100 ml/minute or slower if patient is unable to tolerate this rate of filling or is known to have a neuropathic bladder.
- Fill the bladder with the patient in a supine position.
- Note the first sensation, the normal desire to void, strong desire to void and urgency.
- Aim to fill bladder to between 400 and 500 ml.
- Once the bladder is filled stand patient upright on the floor.
- Encourage patient to cough and bounce on her heels to demonstrate whether sphincter weakness is present.
- Ask patient to void into the flowmeter with rectal and intravesical lines *in situ*.
- Remove all tubes once voiding is complete.
- Give patient a cloth and towel and direct to toilet to wash.
- Give the patient the leaflet entitled 'advice following urodynamic investigations'.

## Troubleshooting

1. If the patient is unable to void pre-test:
   - allow her to void in the toilet outside of the room;
   - continue the test as normal ensuring that any residual urine is recorded on the sheet after the test;
   - document that she was unable to void pre-test.
2. If patient is unable to tolerate 400–500 ml of fluid in her bladder:
   - stop the infusion to see whether the urgency goes away;
   - recommence infusion if urgency diminishes;
   - if the urgency remains, note the volume infused and record on chart.
3. If the patient has a complicated history or has already had surgery to the bladder, there is a possibility that she may have an anatomical abnormality coexisting with bladder dysfunction and videourodynamics should be performed.
   - See procedure above, but fill with radiographic contrast material (urograffin).
   - Check date of LMP. If there is a possibility that she could be pregnant, do a pregnancy test. Document all results and replies.
   - Ensure that all medical staff in the room are wearing a lead coat during imaging.
   - Ensure that the test is videoed and interesting images are put onto film.
4. If the patient has a history of rheumatic fever, aortic valve replacement, then it is essential that they have prophylactic antibiotic cover prior to the test. If this is not possible, then reschedule and ensure that antibiotics have been given.
5. It is important that the machinery is regularly serviced (see manufacturer's guidelines and instructions) and that the transducers are calibrated on a regular basis

# Developing a nurse-led continence service

It is essential before setting up a continence service that the facilities and equipment needed to provide the service are in place.

Equipment needed:

- Assessment form.
- Quiet room for assessment with couch in it.
- Urinalysis dipstix and facilities for sending off samples should an infection be suspected.
- Flow meter for flow rates.
- Bladder scanner to assess residual urines post micturition.
- Advice and information leaflets.

- Access to medical staff for:
  - (a) prescription of medication;
  - (b) referral to other disciplines;
  - (c) addition to the surgical waiting list;
  - (d) advice in more complicated cases.
- Devices such as a perineometer, Neen Pelvic Floor Educators.

## The practitioner

The nurse specialist/continence advisor running the clinics needs to have a qualification or further education in continence assessment and management, and must ensure that s/he is competent in the assessment and management of incontinence.

## Some of the skills needed when assessing continence

- Compassion.
- Time.
- Understanding of the conditions that cause incontinence and their implications.
- Diplomacy.
- Accountability.
- Competency.
- Assertiveness.

# 7 | Menopause

## Management of the menopause

### Definition

The menopause is defined as the permanent cessation of menstruation. Other definitions that are used are:

- The peri-menopause or climacteric is characterized by endocrinological, biological and clinical changes. This can include irregular menstruation although some women do not have this and their periods stop suddenly.
- A woman is defined as post menopausal 12 months after her last natural menstrual period.
- Premature menopause is defined as the menopause occurring under the age of 40 (premature ovarian failure POF).

Within the menopause there are other definitions for the type of menopause:

- Natural – diagnosed after 12 months of amenorrhoea.
- Surgical – removal of the ovaries.
- Induced – normally by radiotherapy, chemotherapy or GnRH analogues. This may be temporary or permanent.

There is a huge variation in the age range of the menopause. In the UK the average age is 51 years old with a range from 45 to 58 years. Women who smoke tend to have an earlier menopause. In general women can therefore, live for 30 years in a post menopausal state.

It is estimated that 75% of women have menopausal symptoms but only 10–20 % receive HRT. It is essential that women receive accurate information about HRT and the menopause in order for them to make an informed choice about whether to take HRT or not. Women with menopausal symptoms can generally be managed by their GP or in well women clinics. However, specialist menopause clinics have a role to play in the management of women with co existing medical conditions, recurrent symptoms on HRT, implant therapy and premature ovarian failure.

### Physiology of the menopause

As the ovaries become unresponsive to FSH the cycles become anovulatory. Follicular development fails and there is no production of oestrogen. The low oestrogen leads to a raised FSH initially followed by a rise in LH. It follows that there is no stimulation of endometrium that leads clinically to amenorrhoea.

Clinical manifestations of the climacteric

- Anovulatory cycles: 3–7% cycles are anovulatory between the ages of 26 and 40 years and this rises to 12–15% between 41 and 51 years:
  (a) reduced fertility;
  (b) erratic menstrual bleeding.
- Increase in FSH: the rise in FSH is gradual and there is a wide fluctuation in the climacteric period;
- onset of menopausal symptoms (see below).

## The menopause clinic

The main aims of a menopause clinic are to maximize the quality of life by reducing symptoms and decreasing the risk of cardiovascular disease and osteoporosis. The decision making process in such clinics is shown in *Figure 7.1*.

Included in this assessment is investigating the women's symptoms and determining if they are true symptoms of the menopause or other symptoms of a different pathology or psychological. It is also of paramount importance to ensure that the women have realistic expectations about treatment with HRT and its duration of treatment. The other aims are to establish positive indications for HRT and specific contraindications.

The clinic should not only be related to giving information and prescribing HRT but also needs to examine other life style changes including:

- stopping smoking;
- regular weight bearing exercise;
- healthy eating, include sufficient calcium;
- correct BMI.

History and examination

- To ascertain the menopausal status LMP and any menopausal symptoms. This can be established within the clinic or by a questionnaire sent to patients prior to the appointment.
- Full past gynaecology, medical and surgical history including any history of hormone dependant malignancies or thromboses/emboli (DVT/PE).
- Special attention to bleeding patterns, identifying anything abnormal and investigating this prior to commencement on HRT.
- Indications for HRT: menopausal symptoms, premature ovarian failure, and osteoporosis risk factors.
- Has the women taken any hormones before i.e. COCP, HRT, and whether she suffered any side effects.

- Her need for contraception.
- Family history of cardiovascular disease (CVD), osteoporosis, DVT, breast cancer, bowel cancer or ovarian cancer.
- Smoking.
- Alcohol.
- Height.
- Weight.
- Blood pressure.
- Pelvic, abdominal and breast examination if clinically indicated in relation to past/current disease, any symptoms or family history.
- The teaching of breast awareness.

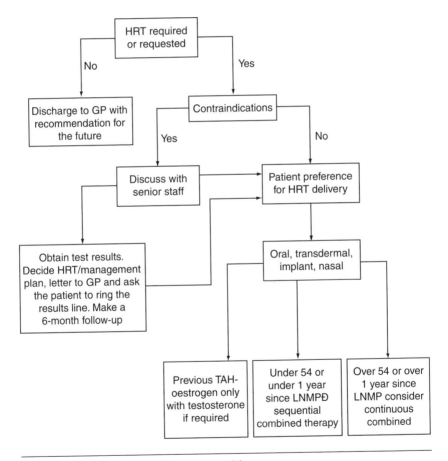

Figure 7.1. **Management of the menopause (1)**

# Short-term menopausal symptoms

Short-term symptoms. These are the most common reasons for women presenting to their doctors and the subsequent prescribing of HRT:

- vasomotor symptoms;
- psychological symptoms;
- urinary and vaginal symptoms.

## Vasomotor symptoms

Hot flushes are periods of inappropriate heat loss that occur in about 75% of women. They start prior to the LMP and increase in incidence in the first year after the last period. They can remain a problem for 5 years in about 25% of women. Each episode lasts for between 2.5 and 3.3 min and vary in frequency from 1 to 2 per week up to 20/day.

Women complain of periods of intense heat, sweating, shivering and tachycardia. At the time of the flushes women can also have faintness, weakness, vertigo, nausea and vomiting, insomnia and palpitations. When they occur at night there is a decrease in rapid eye movement, sleep is disturbed with more frequent waking. This leads to tiredness. Night sweats affect 75% women and can lead to irritability, anxiety, depression, fatigue and inability to concentrate.

The pathophysiology varies from individual to individual. The onset of hot flushes is due to a decrease in the concentration in oestradiol and not the absolute oestradiol levels. They are also linked to changes in plasma levels of adrenaline and noradrenaline, which can cause supraventricular tachycardias, peripheral vasodilatation and anxiousness. There is increasing evidence that serotonin has a role to play in the development of hot flushes.

Untreated hot flushes will cause no long-term harm.

*Treatment of vasomotor symptoms*
- HRT.
- Vitamin E.
- Propanolol, although there is conflicting evidence of the effectiveness of this.
- Clonidine.
- Oil of evening primrose.
- Change in diet/lifestyle.
- Complimentary therapies.
- Decreasing caffeine and alcohol.
- Avoiding hot baths.
- Avoiding trigger foods.
- Decreasing smoking.
- Progestogen. High dose progestogen can be used alone in women with a contraindication to oestrogen in the treatment of hot flushes. As the dose is

high it also offers limited skeletal protection but can carry an increased risk of DVT/PE.

- Selective serotonin re-uptake inhibitors – venlafaxine and paroxetine.

## Psychological symptoms

About 25–50% women suffer with psychological symptoms (Box 7.1).

Many menopausal women complain of deterioration in memory and neurological function, which are often misdiagnosed. The symptoms may vary with the woman's cultural background and if she has a negative perception of the menopause

There is debate as to whether these symptoms are related to a lack of oestrogen or secondary to other symptoms e.g. persistent night sweats lead to poor sleeping that contributes to a reduced concentration span that affects memory and ultimately mood.

They can also be related to external factors such as life changes that occur concurrently with the menopause.

Treatment with HRT may prevent or slow down the progress of Alzheimer's.

| Box 7.1 | Psychological symptoms |
| --- | --- |

- Nervousness
- Anxiety
- Irritability
- Confusion
- Agitation
- Depression
- Loss of libido
- Forgetfulness
- Difficulty in concentration
- Loss of confidence
- Fatigue
- Low self-esteem

## Urinary and vaginal symptoms

Urogential tissue in both the urethra and vagina is oestrogen sensitive and the decline in oestradiol levels leads to symptoms related to a lack of lubrication. In addition the vagina shortens and becomes narrower. This can lead to sexual dysfunction (Box 7.2, 7.3).

Sexual dysfunction is multi-faceted and can be classed as both psychological and urogenital symptoms. There is a role of the lack of oestrogen as a cause for some of the problems that women experience. However, there is also a non-hormonal role, which can involve conflict with partner, insomnia, stress, depression, change of body image and low self-esteem.

Treatment with topical estrogens can make a significant difference to the urogenital symptoms and improve the distress of dyspareunia but some couples may need additional help from a psychosexual counsellor.

| Box 7.2 | Vaginal symptoms |
| --- | --- |

- Infections
- Dyspareunia
- Post-coital bleeding
- Irritation
- Itching
- Decreased libido

| Box 7.3 | Urinary symptoms |
| --- | --- |

- Dysuria
- Frequency
- Urgency
- Post-micturition bleeding
- Urge incontinence
- Stress incontinence

# Long-term menopausal symptoms

Although short-term symptoms of oestrogen deficiency can cause disturbance to the woman's life and functioning it is the effect of long-term oestrogen deficiency that has a greater bearing on both quality and quantity of life.

## Bones and osteoporosis

Bone density is known to decrease with the menopause. Once bone mass is lost it is hard to replace. One in three women and one in 12 men develop osteoporosis. This can only be diagnosed by a bone density scan.

Bone mass peaks in the third decade and slowly declines from then. Following the menopause there is an accelerated loss, which can end with the development of osteoporosis. Not all women develop this and the risk factors are laid out below (*Box 7.4*).

Osteoporosis is characterized by a low bone mass and micro architectural destruction of bone tissue, which can lead to an increased fracture risk particularly of wrists, hips and crush fractures of the spine. It is estimated that fractures cost about £942 million/year.

In the menopause a lack of oestrogen increases the bone turnover and causes an imbalance between re-absorption and formation of bone. Women can loose up to 50% of trabecular bone.

| Box 7.4 | The risk of developing osteoporosis is not related entirely to the menopause as bone mass can be affected by |
|---|---|

- Race
- Sex
- Hereditary factors including a past family history
- Hormonal factors
- Exercise
- Low dietary calcium
- Early menopause < 45 years old
- High intake of alcohol
- Smoking
- Low body weight
- Nulliparity
- Episodes of amenorrhoea
- Sedentary lifestyle
- The long-term use of steroids either oral or inhalers
- Hyperparathyroidism
- Cushing's syndrome
- Other chronic diseases e.g. rheumatoid arthritis

In the treatment of osteoporosis HRT has been shown to improve and stop the decrease of bone density. There are other treatments that can be helpful if the women will not or cannot take HRT:

- Bisphosphonates such as Eitronate and Alendronate. These need to be taken on an empty stomach and can cause gastro-intestinal disturbances.
- SERMS (selective oestrogen receptor modulators) Raloxifene, which has been shown to reduce vertebral fractures although it can cause vasomotor symptoms and has an increased risk of thrombosis. However, it has no adverse affects on breast or endometrial tissue.
- Exercise.

- Calcium and vitamin D.
- Calcitonin.
- Progesterone.
- Parathyroid hormone which can be used with HRT.
- Statins – there is evidence that they may reduce the risk of fracture.

## Heart disease and the menopause

Heart disease is a leading cause of death in women and the role of HRT in preventing this is still controversial. Women who are premenopausal are at less risk due to oestrogen production.

If a women has an early menopause then there is an increased risk of heart disease. After menopause there is a 3.4-fold increase risk. It has been quoted from some studies that there could be up to a 50% reduction in CVD on HRT. However, a recent study has contradicted this in women who are on continuous combined HRT and are at high risk of developing CVD. Further studies are awaited to clarify this controversy. Currently there is no evidence to suggest that low risk women should stop taking HRT, particularly if they are on cyclical or oestrogen only preparations. Women on continuous combined preparations should be given an individualized risk based on their past medical and family history, and advised whether or not to continue on HRT or change preparations according to this risk assessment.

## Blood tests and investigations

- FSH is only of value if the diagnosis of the climacteric from the symptoms is in doubt.
- LH, oestradiol, progestogen and testosterone are of no value in assessing ovarian function. Oestradiol is only of benefit in examining therapeutic levels of hormones in non-oral routes of administration.
- TFT (free T4 and TSH) can be used if the presenting symptoms are lethargy, weight gain, hair loss and flushes if the diagnosis of the menopause is in doubt especially in relation to non-response to HRT.
- 24-Hour urine for catecholamines, 5-hydroxindolacetic acid and methylhistamines to exclude the rarer causes of hot flushes such as phaeochromocytoma, carcinoid syndrome and mastocytosis.
- Any investigations that are needed for either the family history or medical history. Thyroid, clotting screen, lipid profile, hormone profile, cervical smears and mammogram.
- Bone density scan especially if high risk – untreated menopause, POF, steroids, eating disorders, and height loss. Bone density may also be useful in helping women in a decision of whether to take HRT.

## Treatments

There are two main classes of treatment that will be described more fully in the next section of this chapter.

Hormonal

- Oestrogen alone.
- Oestrogen plus progesterone.
- Progesterone alone.

Non-hormonal

- Lifestyle.
- Medication.
- Alternative therapies.

With all treatments including HRT it is important to stress the realistic time frame for resolution of symptoms. It can take up to 3/12 to resolve vasomotor symptoms. If this has not happened then the staff should be checking that patients are compliant with the medication, taking it properly and that the delivery route is correct for them.

It can take up to 6/12 to combat urogenital symptoms and a year for psychological symptoms to resolve. During this time the woman needs support and guidance and to persevere with the treatment. *Figure 7.2* gives a suggestion for follow-up of patients who choose to take HRT.

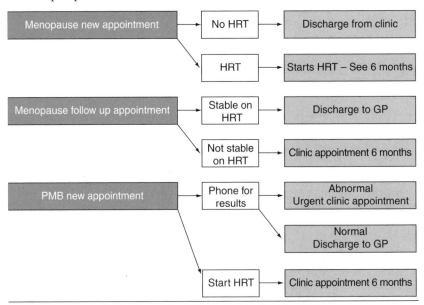

**Figure 7.2. Management of the menopause (2)**

# HRT

In counselling women with regard to HRT it is important to give an explanation of the menopause, the long-term benefits of HRT, risks of HRT and side effects.

The long-term benefits of HRT have been discussed in the pervious section in relation to osteoporosis and heart disease. There is also thought to be emerging evidence that use of HRT can help prevent or slow down the progress of Alzheimer's.

## Contraception

Around the menopause it is difficult to assess when fertility stops as cycles continue and may be anovulatory but a few cycles will result in ovulation leading to a risk of conception. If women are not taking HRT then the advice can be given that if they are over 50 years old they should continue to use contraception until they are at least 1 year after their LMP, if they are under 50 then this should be 2 years. The difficulties arise when women are taking HRT as this will not be known. Women should be warned that HRT is not a contraceptive and that they should ensure that they are using a suitable method of contraception.

## Advantages of HRT

- Decrease of hot flushes.
- Improvement in vaginal dryness.
- Employed in conservative management of urinary continence.
- Increase bone mass.
- Effecting mood, cognition.
- Increase quality of life.

## Risks of HRT

Thrombosis

There is a risk of thrombosis in taking HRT. This risk is theoretically low rising from 1/10000 to 3/10000 if she has no other risk factors. Risk factors that can be identified in her history include:

- cardiovascular disease – valve disease, atrial fibrillation;
- massive obesity;
- history of thrombosis;
- history of thrombosis on the COCP or in pregnancy;
- strong family history of thrombosis.

Breast cancer

A woman in the UK has a lifetime risk of breast cancer of 10%. Women who have never used HRT aged 50–70 years old have a risk of 45/1000. The risk of breast cancer is increased on HRT in addition to the background risk that a women may have in relation to family history and other medical factors. HRT use confers a similar risk year on year similar to that of a late menopause (*Box 7.5*). This increased risk does not apply to women who experience POF suggesting that it is the lifetime exposure to oestrogen that confers the risk. If a woman has a specific family history she should be referred for genetic counselling prior to the commencement on HRT to establish her individual risk.

| Box 7.5 | Rates of the increase in breast cancer in women age 50–70 using HRT are |
| --- | --- |

- 45/1000 up to 47/1000 with 5 years use
- 51/1000 up to 57/1000 with 10 years use
- 57/1000 up to 69/1000 with 15 years use.

But mortality rates are lower in women who develop breast cancer while on HRT.

## HRT types

There are many different types of HRT and approximately 50 are licensed in the UK. These are broadly defined by the contents of the product (*Box 7.6*) and the mode of delivery (*Box 7.7*).

| Box 7.6 | Contents of HRT |
| --- | --- |

- Oestrogen only
- Sequential combined
- Continuous combined
- Tibolone
- Testosterone

- Progesterone is needed for women who have not had a hysterectomy to prevent endometrial hyperplasia.
- About 80% women with a uterus take oral therapy and 15% have patches.
- Women who have had a hysterectomy can be given oestrogen only in any of the delivery forms below (*Box 7.7*).
- Women in the peri-menopause are normally given sequential monthly bleed therapy.
- Women who are post menopausal can safely have continuous combined therapy eliminating the need for the monthly withdrawal bleed.
- If women are changing from sequential combined therapy to continuous combined it can be difficult to know when they can safely do this without encountering irregular bleeding. By the age of 54, 80% of women will be post menopausal and can be safely changed. If a woman has 6 months previous amenorrhoea or a raised FSH in her 40s and has been on HRT for several years continuous therapy can be tried. When changing or starting on continuous therapy women should be warned to expect irregular bleeding for the first 4–6 months. Endometrial assessment should be undertaken if the bleeding becomes heavy, persists after 6 months or after a significant period of amenorrhoea.

| Box 7.7 | Mode of delivery |
| --- | --- |

- Oral therapy
- Transdermal therapy
- Subcutaneous therapy
- Vaginal
- Nasal
- Intra uterine

## Existing medical conditions and the relationship with HRT

There are no absolute contraindications to HRT from a past medical history but it is important to consider each individual's relative risk and present it accurately to the patient. Liaison with the patient's specialist or referral to a specialist is recommended for some pre-existing medical conditions (*see Box 7.8*).

| Box 7.8 | Relative risks of pre-existing medical conditions |
|---|---|
| **Condition** | **Comments** |
| Angina | No contraindication |
| Asthma | HRT OK if stable – oestrogen may improve problem but progesterone may make it worse |
| Benign breast disease | No contraindication |
| Abnormal smears, cancer of the cervix | No contraindication |
| Depression | No contraindication, progesterone may exacerbate problem |
| Diabetes | No contraindication – if seen in specialist service, consider Transdermal therapy |
| Endometriosis | No contraindication – can cause re activation of disease, consider continuous combined therapy or tibalone even after TAH to suppress deposits. |
| Epilepsy | No contraindication – consider Transdermal |
| Hypertension | No contraindication. Blood pressure may rise on conjugated equine oestrogen |
| Migraines/headaches | No contraindication – discontinue if problems worsen. If cyclical try continuous combined |
| Ovarian cancer | No contraindication |
| Renal failure | No contraindication – may cause fluid retention |
| Sickle cell | No contraindication |
| Smoking | No contraindication |
| Stroke | No contraindication |
| Thyroid disease | No contraindication – thyroxine will need to be monitored. |
| Fibroids | No contraindication – may enlarge and will require monitoring of size and amount of bleeding |
| Endometrial hyperplasia | Can be corrected by HRT |
| Gall bladder disease | Advise Transdermal therapy |
| Lactose intolerance | Not oral therapy |
| Liver disease | Check LFT's prior to treatment – advise Transdermal |
| SLE | May deteriorate on HRT |
| Breast and ovarian cancer | Treated patients should be seen by specialist clinic. Patients with family history need counselling and genetic referral. |
| Endometrial cancer | Complete surgical resection – HRT under guidance<br>Incomplete – can have high dose progesterone |
| DVT/PE | ? Referral for thrombophilia screen – advise transdermal HRT |

## Contents of HRT

### Oestrogen

Oestrogens are available in natural and synthetic forms. Synthetic forms are not used for HRT and it is the natural oestrogens in the form of oestradiol, oestrone and oestriol, which are derived mainly from soya beans and yams. Conjugated equine oestrogen is made from pregnant horses' urine and is also in this natural category.

### Progestrogens

There are different types of progestrogen used in different preparations. Within the clinic it is important to know which progestrogens are in which preparations and which side effects they can cause so that treatment can be tailored to women's individual needs. The most commonly used progestrogens are:

- Norethisterone;
- Levonorgestrol;
- Dydrogesterone;
- Medroxyprogesterone acetate.

The last two are less androgenic and can decrease acne and greasy skin.

Progestogens are given for 10–14 days of a 28-day cycle in peri-menopausal women. Sequential therapy should give a mean bleed of 3–7 days. Most women experience a regular monthly bleed although some will have no bleeding (20%). Between 57 and 91% of women experience scheduled bleeding after the withdrawal of the progesterone. If women are peri-menopausal and wish to have bleed-free therapy then they can consider the IUS.

In women who are 1 year post menopausal a continuous low dose progestogen can be given alongside the oestrogen which will prevent endometrial hyperplasia. The women experience no monthly bleeding. However, some women will experience irregular bleeding in the first few months with 75% achieving amenorrhoea in 6 months. This rate increases the longer the time the woman is from her LMP. If women experience vaginal bleeding after a period of amenorrhoea this needs to be investigated. Continuous therapy keeps the endometrium atrophic. It has been suggested that it is safer for the endometrium than sequential HRT in post menopausal women.

Progestogen can also be given every 3 months, which still maintains endometrial protection and is particularly useful if women experience severe progestogen side effects. Women who have had an endometrial ablation still need to have progestogen in their HRT.

## Side effects

As with all medication there can be side effects with HRT. It is therefore of paramount importance when starting women on HRT to counsel about these and to warn women to be realistic. HRT is not a quick fix, one size fits all preparation.

Side effects are common in the first few weeks and normally resolve after 3 months

If side effects persist it is important to establish if they are related to the oestrogen (*Box 7.9*) or the progestogen (*Box 7.10*).

| Box 7.9 Oestrogen related side effects | |
|---|---|
| • Breast tenderness | • Nipple sensitivity |
| • Nausea | • Headaches |
| • Leg cramps | • Dyspepsia |
| • Bloating | |

They usually resolve but if they do not consider changing to a different oestrogen.

They can be worse if the woman is more than 5 years post menopause and this can be minimized by starting with a very low dose.

Otherwise observe the patient and wait, reduce the dose or change the mode of delivery.

| Box 7.10 Progestogen related side effects | | |
|---|---|---|
| • Fluid retention, bloating | • Mood changes | • Dysmenorrhoea |
| • Breast tenderness | • Depression | • Clumsiness |
| • Abdominal cramps | • Headaches | • Bleeding problems |
| • Anxiety | • Acne | |

These can be reduced or alleviated by changing or adjusting the type of progesterone (testosterone or progesterone derivatives.) or by changing the route of the frequency of administration.

Consider the use of the progestogen only IUS if neither oral or transdermal progesterone is tolerated.

## Mode of delivery

Oral therapy

The tablets can be oestrogen only, sequential with 12 days of combined progestogen and oestrogen or continuous therapy with both oestrogen and progesterone. These are tablets that are absorbed by the gut, and pass into the hepatic portal circulation where they are 98% metabolized on the first pass through the liver. Owing to this effect tablets contain larger doses of oestrogen and progesterone than other methods and this can cause nausea.

Advantages:
• cheap;
• convenient;
• familiar form to take medication.

Disadvantages:
• disrupts the ratio of oestradiol to oestrone;
• need compliance from the patient;
• can cause nausea;

- not to be used in patients with: liver problems, hypertension, hypertriglyceridaemia, DVT, GI problems.

The levels of circulating hormones obtained are variable and they may not control symptoms. Tibolone is included in this oral group. Although not a true HRT it contains estrogenic- progestogenic- and androgenic-like properties that reduce hot flushes, increase mood and libido and do not induce bleeding if women are 1 year past the menopause. It is also protective of bones.

## Transdermal

This is given in the form of a patch or a gel, which means that the hormones are absorbed through the skin. This therapy gives better hormonal levels and sometimes improved symptom control. Patches are applied to the thighs, buttocks or abdomen and need changing either once or twice a week.

**Advantages:**
- no need to take tablets;
- normal ratio of oestradiol to oestrone;
- avoids the liver;
- can be perceived as natural;
- it is a delivery mode of choice in patients who are diabetic, have liver problems, digestive problems and those on some medications.

**Disadvantages:**
- difference in degree of adhesion in different patients;
- can cause side effects especially skin irritation;
- it is a visual reminder to the women that she is menopausal;
- compliance relies on women changing patches.

## Implants

Implants of oestrogen and/or testosterone are given into the subcutaneous fat of the abdomen or buttocks on a 6-monthly basis. The levels of oestrogen given are generally higher than in tablets or patches.

**Advantages:**
- gives good control of symptoms;
- minimum need for compliance from the women;
- given twice a year;
- avoids the liver;
- can give testosterone to relieve libido reduction;
- cheap;
- convenient for the woman especially in women after TAH.

**Disadvantages:**
- need to be inserted by a health care professional;

- involves a minor procedure;
- prolonged use can give rise to tachyphylaxsis – oestrogen levels are within normal limits but they experience symptoms of oestrogen withdrawal;
- the effects of the oestrogen can last up to 2 years so in women who have a uterus, they need to continue progesterone for 2 years after the last implant.

### Vaginal

Local therapy can be given to women who have atrophic vaginitis and/or urethritis without the systemic effects from HRT. It can be given in the form of creams, pessaries or vaginal tablets. These are normally used 4–5 times a week for 2–3 weeks then reduced to twice a week for 2–3 months, with some women repeating this for a few weeks as a maintenance dose.

A new vaginal ring can also be used but this is systemic therapy and requires additional progesterone if the women has an intact uterus.

**Advantages:**
- no bleeding;
- effective for urogential symptoms;
- can be used in conjunction with HRT for persistent urogential symptoms;
- convenient.

**Disadvantages:**
- messy;
- can be difficult to use in the elderly;
- regulation can be difficult.

### Nasal

Intranasal oestrogen is rapidly absorbed via the nasal mucous to increase plasma concentrations to reach a maximum 10–30 minutes after inhalation. This then returns to the post menopausal levels 12 hours later. A dose of 300 ug is as effective as 2 mg of oral oestrogen. There are currently trials underway to look at continuous combined nasal HRT.

## Alternatives to HRT

- For hot flushes: Clonidine, anti-hypertensives 50–75 µg BD. These can reduce flushes in about 30% women. They do however have some side effects: dry mouth, dizziness, fatigue and nausea.
- For atrophic vaginitis: lubrication creams.
- Osteoporosis: biphosphonate etidronate, Alendronate
- SERMs – work on specific tissues, tamoxifen but adverse effects on endometrium (6 × increase risk of endometrial cancer) raloxifene is better but there is an increase in vasomotor symptoms better in post menopausal women with a high risk of osteoporosis.

- Phytoestrogens come from plants and have a similar structure to oestrogen. The main ones are isoflavones from soya and clover and ligans from flax and cereals. In countries that have a high amount of phytoestrogen in their diet there is a decrease in menopausal symptoms, CVD, osteoporosis, breast cancer, colon cancer and endometrial cancer.
- Ginseng has some oestrogen-like properties.
- Black Cosh can be beneficial for some menopausal symptoms.
- St John's wort can be beneficial in depression, increasing psychological symptoms.
- DHEA.

## Compliance on HRT

Thirty-nine percent of women will discontinue HRT due to side effects.

Compliance is a large issue in HRT. This is where building a therapeutic relationship with women can be of help, it is also helpful to ensure that women have adequate knowledge and have made an informed choice to start on HRT. Compliance varies from woman to woman. Women generally stop HRT due to side effects or because they do not believe the advice that they have been given. They need to be motivated and have a general discussion about future health problems in relation to initial side effects. Discontinuation may arise from any of the following:

- worried by risks;
- not enough information;
- incomplete knowledge;
- weight gain although this is perceived and studies have demonstrated that women on and off HRT gain weight and change body shape at the same rate when going through the menopause;
- side effects.

Compliance can be affected by:

- involving women in the decision making process;
- discussing unrealistic expectations;
- clear and personalized explanation of the benefits, risks and duration of treatment;
- written information;
- follow-up;
- the gender of the prescriber.

## Bleeding on HRT

Women on sequential HRT should have regular withdrawal bleeds that are not too heavy or painful. Some women have amenorrhoea and this does not need investigation. Abnormal bleeding on HRT is relatively rare and includes PCB and IMB.

Causes of bleeding include:

- polyps;
- submucosal fibroids;
- uterine malignancy;
- bleeding on continuous therapy, check post menopausal and on correct therapy. If within first 6 months observe, if persists investigate;
- idiopathic – this can be reduced by changing oestrogen, progestrogen or route of administration;
- spontaneous ovarian activity;
- endometrial hyperplasia;
- unscheduled bleeding may be due to the woman's underlying cycle. Beginning the progestrogen 12 days prior to the expected start of menstruation can reduce this.

Women should be investigated if they have any abnormal bleeding. This should be performed in a one-stop clinic environment where there is access to ultrasound, endometrial biopsy and hysteroscopy if needed.

An endometrial thickness of >8 mm in a woman on HRT or any irregularity should be considered abnormal and a hysteroscopy and endometrial biopsy performed.

If investigations have been performed and are normal then the following can be tried.

- If the bleeding is heavy, painful, starts too early or is prolonged the progestogen can be increased or changed.
- Spotting early in the cycle, increase the oestrogen.
- If breakthrough bleeding is a persistent problem then it needs to be investigated. This can be due to poor compliance, drug interactions, GI upset or stress.

# Management of the menopause clinic

## Referral

Letters of referral should be managed similarly to other clinics. A menopause questionnaire (*Figure 7.3*) should be included in the appointment letter that should be filled in and brought to the clinic. However, in some instances the patient may be referred directly to the nurse practitioner or to the minor procedures clinic or specialist bleeding on HRT clinic if demand is high enough. The circumstances include the following

Directly to nurse practitioner

- Referral to clinic following a hysterectomy where an implant has been inserted.
- Referral from a general clinic or GP for a woman who is well established on HRT implants.

This questionnaire will help you to gain the most from your consultation. On subsequent visits it will help to assess if the treatment given is appropriate for you.

Please tick the appropriate box.

|  | Yes | No |
|---|---|---|
| 1. Are you currently taking HRT | ☐ | ☐ |
| 2. If yes what? | | |
| 3. If yes are you getting symptom relief | ☐ | ☐ |

**Do you currently have:**

| | Yes | No |
|---|---|---|
| 1. Hot flushes during the day | ☐ | ☐ |
| 2. Night sweats | ☐ | ☐ |
| 3. Inability to sleep | ☐ | ☐ |
| 4. Headaches | ☐ | ☐ |
| 5. Tiredness | ☐ | ☐ |
| 6. Loss of energy | ☐ | ☐ |
| 7. General aches and pains | ☐ | ☐ |
| 8. General itchiness | ☐ | ☐ |
| 9. Emotional problems | ☐ | ☐ |
| 10. Panic attacks | ☐ | ☐ |
| 11. Palpitations | ☐ | ☐ |
| 12. Bladder problems | ☐ | ☐ |
| 13. Sexual problems | ☐ | ☐ |
| 14. Vaginal dryness | ☐ | ☐ |
| 15. Loss of memory and concentration | ☐ | ☐ |

When was your first day of your last menstrual period? Date:

If within the last 6 months, how many days do you bleed for?

How often do you bleed?

**Your periods.**

| | Yes | No |
|---|---|---|
| 1. Are your periods lighter? | ☐ | ☐ |
| 2. Are your periods erratic? | ☐ | ☐ |
| 3. Are your periods heavier? | ☐ | ☐ |
| 4. Are your periods painful? | ☐ | ☐ |
| 5. Do you bleed in-between periods? | ☐ | ☐ |
| 6. Do you bleed after intercourse? | ☐ | ☐ |
| 7. If you are taking bleed free HRT have you had any bleeding? | ☐ | ☐ |

What do you wish to discuss in the consultation?

Do you have any particular worries?

**Figure 7.3.** Menopausal symptom assessment

To Minor Procedures/Rapid Access/Bleeding on HRT clinic

- Women with abnormal bleeding whilst on HRT, this may include
  (a) IMB;
  (b) PCB;
  (c) heavy cyclical bleeding;
  (d) painful bleeding.

## Management in clinic

A suitably experienced doctor must be available to the nurse practitioner in order for her/him to discuss any problems that may arise during the consultation and/or to prescribe the implants. It is hoped that in the near future nurse practitioners will be able to prescribe implants and HRT if there is no change in therapy required. In the event that the dose or nature of the HRT needs to be changed then a senior doctor should be consulted regardless of whether the patient is seen by a nurse or junior doctor.

The nurse should collate investigations such as lipid profiles, bone densitometry, oestradiol levels. A telephone number with a time that is convenient to the nurse should be given to the patients so that the results can be given direct to the patient together with a management plan. A letter should subsequently be sent to the GP (*Figure 7.1*).

### First visit

The appointment should be 30 minutes long. The clinician should take a full history using the menopause questionnaire and examination with an assessment of risk factors for the individual woman for taking HRT. There should be sufficient time in the appointment to fully inform the patient of the advantages and disadvantages of HRT, the types of HRT available. The choice of going on HRT is largely the decision of the patient but the doctor or nurse plays a crucial role in making sure the information is specific to the individual patient with a particular emphasis on the advantages and risks based on the severity of her menopausal symptoms, her risk of developing cardiovascular disease and osteoporosis, her risk of side effects, particularly breast cancer and thrombosis.

If the patient decides not to take HRT she should be referred back to her GP. The letter should include an assessment of the risk for the patient of developing osteoporosis and a recommendation for future bone densitometry measurements/need for alternative therapy. If she decides to take HRT she should be offered a follow-up appointment in 6 months time.

### Follow-up

The follow-up visit should include a review of the patient's symptoms based on the original assessment. A repeat questionnaire can be given before seeing the patient to establish whether there has been an improvement. If the patient is happy with the treatment she should be discharged back to the GP. If her symptoms persist or she complains of side effects then further discussion about the available types of HRT should take place and the treatment changed or stopped. A further appointment should be given for 6 months.

## Nurse-led menopause clinics

The management of women using implants as HRT is one area that can be undertaken by a nurse practitioner or consultant nurse as an independent practitioner. To reach the point of independent practise the following arrangements need to be made:

- The nurse must be trained to take a full medical, surgical and gynaecological history. S/he should be able to advise on a full breast examination and take a cervical smear.
- The nurse practitioner should have a full and in-depth understanding of the menopause, be able to discuss the advantages and disadvantages of HRT, the drugs administered, the various delivery systems and any side effects that may occur.
- A standing order for the implants needs to made with pharmacy which will only be valid for women who receive the same dose of implant at each visit.
- The nurse practitioner should have undergone training to be competent at the insertion of implants. This will involve observing at least 20 implants and then inserting at least 15 implants under direct supervision until the practitioner and assessor feel that competence is achieved. After this initial period indirect supervision should be continued until both the trainer and trainee are sure that competency has been achieved.
- If the practitioner feels that the dose needs to be altered s/he will discuss this with the relevant doctor and obtain a prescription.

### Clinic visit

The main aim of the visit is to assess whether the woman is happy to continue with the implant and whether this is the most appropriate treatment option for her.

- The woman is assessed on arrival:
  (a) in regard to the implants i.e. if hysterectomy when and for what reason;
  (b) past medical and surgical history;
  (c) allergies;
  (d) medication;
  (e) blood pressure;
  (f) self-breast examination and mammogram;
  (g) bone density scan if appropriate;
  (h) smoking/alcohol intake;
  (i) exercise;
  (j) weight.

- If the woman has not had a hysterectomy the nurse should check when she last bled and for any history of abnormal bleeding. If there have been any problems the woman should be referred to the one-stop diagnostic clinic.
- Check that cervical smears are up to date and perform this if needed.
- Check that the woman has a supply of progestogen and is taking it as prescribed if she has a uterus.
- Assess whether the woman has had adequate symptom control since her last implant. If she is having significant symptoms more than one month prior to her 6-monthly appointment a serum oestradiol level should be measured. If the level is below 300 pmol/l then she may require an increased dose, at levels higher than this she can be offered low dose oestradiol patches instead of an implant.
- Assess whether the woman has had any side effects.
- Discuss with the woman the reasons for HRT, her expectations and whether implants remain the most suitable therapy for her. Support this with written information.
- Have up to date research-backed information about the risks of endometrial and breast cancer and be able to fully discuss this with women placing it into an approprate context
- Be able to discuss the fears women have regarding weight gain, risk of thrombosis and talk about any unrealistic expectations that they may have.
- Be able to use the opportunity for general health education reducing/stopping smoking, increasing exercise, eating a balanced diet.
- Be able if required to discuss non-hormonal/alternative methods of controlling menopause symptoms or be able to find the information that a women requests.

## Insertion of hormone implants

- Prepare the patient.
- Examine the abdomen for previous scars and choose site for the implant.
- Clean the skin.
- Infiltrate the skin with ligocaine.
- When this is effective make an incision 5 mm to allow the trocar through.
- Insert trocar with cannula through the incision.
- Pinching the abdominal fat push trocar through horizontally avoiding the rectus sheath and muscle.
- Remove the sharp cannula inside the hollow trocar and insert implant(s) through this.

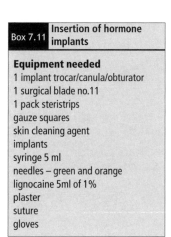

Box 7.11 | **Insertion of hormone implants**

**Equipment needed**
1 implant trocar/canula/obturator
1 surgical blade no.11
1 pack steristrips
gauze squares
skin cleaning agent
implants
syringe 5 ml
needles – green and orange
lignocaine 5ml of 1%
plaster
suture
gloves

- Using the obturator push implants through the trocar and into the subcutaneous fat layer.
- Remove trocar while applying pressure to the wound.
- Apply pressure to the wound.
- If minimal bleeding then apply steristrips and a plaster/gauze and tape
- If necessary a stitch can be inserted.

Nurse practitioners are more than able after adequate training to undertake a caseload of patients. They can take the woman's history and explore issues relating to HRT and the menopause. With further training nurse practitioners and nurse consultants can undertake the management of women with bleeding problems on HRT by being trained to do transvaginal ultrasound and hysteroscopy.

# Roles and Training of Outpatients Staff

# 8 | Roles and Training of Outpatients Staff

## Role of the clinic clerk

The clinic clerk's role within the unit is integral to the patient journey. They are the front-line staff where first impressions are made and can set the scene for the patient experience. If the clerk has little or no understanding of the service provided and their role within that service, then the patient can become frustrated and in extreme cases lose confidence in the care provided.

When a new clerk starts their job they should have:

- 2 weeks' induction where they are supernumerary.
- Clear line management.
- A clear understanding of their role within the unit.
- Named consultant clinics for which they are responsible.
- Access to IT/information services relevant to their role.

As part of the multidisciplinary team the clerk should have:

- Interpersonal skills.
- Customer care skills.
- A good working relationship with the consultant team.
- A forum for expressing their views/ideas for change or improvement.
- Access to training and development that is current and ongoing.
- An ongoing system of appraisal.
- Up to date knowledge of national and local standards, targets and initiatives.

If the clerk has the tools to do their job effectively the patient journey can be seamless. If we refer back to the flow diagram for the management of referral letters (Chapter 1) the clerk has a part to play from the minute the referral is received within the department through to the patient discharge from clinic. The tasks performed by the clinic clerk include the following:

## Referral process

- Receiving, opening and stamping the referral letter.
- Booking the patient onto the hospital's registration mainframe if not done centrally.
- Booking the appointment and generating the appointment letter.
- Sending the appointment letter and investigation forms to the patient or to the relevant department.

- Booking of interpreters.
- Booking of transport.
- Answering queries from the patients and making any necessary changes.

## Before clinic

- Getting all the notes from medical records.
- Registering the arrival of the notes in the department.
- Checking and obtaining any results and filing them.
- Ensuring that all referral letters are filed in the correct notes for new patients.
- Printing out a list of patients and appointment times for the nursing and medical staff.

## During clinic

- Registering arrival of patients and noting the time of arrival.
- Making follow-up appointments.
- Obtaining any missing results.
- Answering patients queries and referring them on to other members of the team as appropriate.

## After clinic

- Returning the notes to medical records if this is not the responsibility of the secretary.
- Filing the approved results when checked by the senior staff.

The clerk is crucial to the efficient running of the clinic and needs to be valued in this role by all members of staff (see *Fig. 8.1*).

# Role of the gynaecology secretary

The role of the clinic secretary is an important part of the multidisciplinary team. Like the clerk, they are integral to the patient journey through the department within the outpatient setting through to discharge from the ward.

Their role is as follows:

- The link between the referrer, patient and consultant team.
- Consultant team administrative support.

When a new secretary starts their job they should have:

- 2 weeks' induction where they are supernumerary.
- Clear line management.

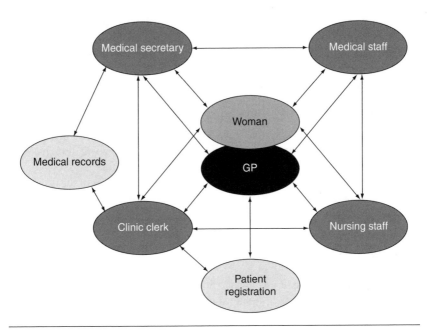

**Figure 8.1. Inter-communication of stakeholders in gynaecology outpatients**

- A clear understanding of their role within the unit.
- Named consultant clinics.
- Access to IT/information services relevant to their role.

As part of the multidisciplinary team the secretary should have:

- Interpersonal skills.
- Customer care skills.
- Named consultant teams.
- Amspar training or equivalent.
- Typing speeds of 50 wpm minimum.
- An ability to prioritize workloads.
- Enough knowledge to highlight to their consultant teams an urgent result.
- The confidence to bring information to the attention of a clinician for action.
- A forum for expressing their views/ideas for change or improvement.
- Access to training and development that is current and ongoing.
- An ongoing system of appraisal.
- Up to date knowledge of national and local standards, targets and iniatives.

The clinic secretary is often the lynchpin for the consultant clinic along with the named clerk. For that consultant team they are the personnel who can access all the information for the patient and relay that information on through the system. Their role within the communication process both internally and externally is paramount to the seamless service an outpatient service needs to provide to meet the demands of a modern, ever changing service.

As new technology is introduced and refined within the NHS the role of the clinic secretary will change. Audio typing will become as rare as shorthand is now. The developments within the EPR (Electronic Patient Record) that will generate a letter for GPs and other referrers at source from the data set provided, will negate the need for dictation following clinic. Voice-activated technology will also challenge traditional secretarial roles. The technology is there and as history has shown developments are slow to start but quickly gain momentum. Secretaries of the future will take more of a PA/administrative role within the consultant team liaising with all the relevant departments and personnel and troubleshooting for their team.

## Role of nursing staff

For the smooth running of any gynaecology clinic it is important that there is a core of dedicated outpatient nursing staff. The numbers and grades of staff will depend on the size and the frequency of clinics. The following sections will outline the different roles that nursing staff have to play within the clinic.

Of paramount importance, as in all nursing, is that the staff have excellent communication skills, not only with the patients but also with the whole team, clerks, secretaries and medical staff. It follows on from this that staff need to be aware of the important role that all of the outpatient staff play in providing care to the patients and work in a multi professional team.

All staff should have an idea of what the department is trying to achieve and their role within it.

In order for nurses to undertake and function in their role it is important that they have all, regardless of grade undertake the following education or training:

- Phlebotomy and cannulation.
- Principles of infection control and decontamination of instruments.
- The handling of complaints and customer care.
- Undertaking baseline observations.
- How to chaperone and assist in procedures.
- Annual fire, resuscitation and manual handling updates.
- Management of clinic sessions.
- Up to date knowledge of national and local standards.
- Basic IT skills to undertake finding of results.
- Identify chronic conditions, which could impact on women's health.
- Recognize the impact that psychological, social and cultural factors can have on the well-being of women.

- Aware of the need for accurate record keeping.
- Communicate effectively with clients, their families and colleagues.
- Maintain the rights of the client/family regarding confidentiality including the Data Protection Act.
- Demonstrate a flexible approach to the delivery of care.
- Be able to set up a minor procedures and general gynaecology clinic.
- Assessment for admission of patients.

These are minimum requirements for all staff and further education and training will need to be identified in appraisals. This training can be in the form of formal courses but is most likely to be in the form of informal training undertaken in the clinic. To undertake these there needs to be an identified sister/senior staff nurse who is in charge of the nursing staff in clinic.

The traditional role of the nurse in outpatients includes:

- Preparation of the clinic rooms.
- Chaperoning and assisting the medical staff.
- Acting as an advocate for the patient.
- Providing information to the patients.
- Informing the patients of how the clinic is running.
- Answering clinical queries on the phone and referring on as appropriate.
- Keeping the clinic well stocked with instruments, relevant paperwork, patient information leaflets.

## Health care assistants (HCA)

Within all clinic settings there needs to be a balance of staff at different grades and abilities. It is therefore essential that there is adequate provision of HCA within the clinics.

They should be responsible for:

- The setting up of the clinic and the clearing of the rooms at the end of each session in conjunction with the qualified staff.
- Undertaking phlebotomy and observations.
- Communicating with patients.
- Liaising with the admissions staff if the department is using patient agreed bookings.
- Assisting in the one-stop clinic.
- Finding results.
- Chaperoning.

This is not an exact list of the duties of the HCA and can be modified according to the grade and training that the have received (see Job Description HCA).

# 1. JOB DETAILS

**JOB TITLE:**          Health Care Assistant

**GRADE:**          B Grade

# 2. JOB PURPOSE

The Clinical Support Worker is a key member of the gynaecology team and works under the direction of qualified nurses assisting in meeting patient's physical, psychological and social needs. The post holder helps with the maintenance of a safe, comfortable, quiet, clean environment for patients, staff and visitors and will assist in performing administrative and clerical duties.

The post holder is expected to work across sites in the gynaecology ward, the early pregnancy assessment unit and outpatient clinics.

# 3. CLINICAL

3.1.  To assist with the running of outpatient and colposcopy clinics.

3.2.  To act as a chaperone in the outpatient clinics.

3.3.  To assist in the preparation of the clinic environment, including replenishing the equipment in clinic rooms and monitoring stock levels.

3.4.  To assist in the Minor Procedures and Colposcopy clinics. To help set up the clinics, assist the nurse and doctor with the procedure. To ensure that patients safety is maintained.

3.5.  To ensure that all equipment is cleaned, correctly maintained and sterilized in accordance with outpatient protocols.

3.6.  Assists with making beds and cleaning bed areas. Prepares bed areas for new admissions. Assists women with hygiene needs. Assists patients with mobilization.

3.7.  To assist in the smooth running of outpatient clinics, welcoming patients to appropriate seating areas and ensuring appropriate results are in the case notes.

3.8.  Escorts patients, at the discretion of the qualified nurse, within/between hospitals and/or departments.

3.9.  Takes patients pulse, blood pressure and temperature and records on appropriate chart. Reports readings to qualified nurse.

3.10. To undertake phlebotomy, once trained.

3.11. Tests urine of designated patients. Reports results to the qualified nurse and takes urine sample as appropriate.

3.12. Assists in preparing patients for procedures/investigations.

3.13. Communicates with patients and is aware of the general needs of good communication.

3.14. Answers telephone, relays and records messages in an accurate manner.

3.15. Assists with the maintenance, cleaning and storage of equipment. Assists with the cleaning of storage areas.

3.16. Assists with the safe-keeping of patients property and valuables.

3.17. Assists in the reception of new patients and visitors. Orientate to given area. Offers and prepares light refreshments where appropriate.

3.18. Internal rotation to work in outpatients, early pregnancy unit and on the gynaecology ward when necessary to meet the needs of the service.

3.19. Carries out other appropriate activities at the direction of the qualified nurse.

## 4. EDUCATIONAL

4.1.  Works with allocated mentor.

4.2.  Identifies learning needs and agrees objectives with mentor.

4.3.  Accepts responsibility for keeping up to date.

## 5. CLERICAL

5.1.  Completes documentation of patients on admission and discharge to the ward and completes appropriate documentation in relation to gynaecology outpatients and the early pregnancy unit. Keeping notes in order, replenishing continuation sheets etc.

5.2.  Admitting patients. Fill out patient information sheet. Liaise with nursing staff regarding their completion of the nursing assessment.

5.3.  Assist in the clerical work required according to the need in the various rotational areas.

5.4.  Liaise and direct visitors in a polite and friendly manner.

## 6. COMMUNICATION

6.1.  Develops positive relationships with all members of the interdisciplinary team.

6.2.  Ensures all patients and visitors are treated in a kind and courteous manner.

6.3.  Maintains privacy of patient.

6.4.  Ensures patients are informed of delays.

6.5.  Ensures patients know where other departments are situated.

6.6.  Reports any complaints to the co-ordinating nurse and assists in any investigation of the same.

6.7.  Acts as chaperone as necessary.

6.8  Answers telephone courteously, respecting patient confidentiality.

# 7. HEALTH AND SAFETY

7.1.   Reports any accidents/incidents to a member of the nursing team.

7.2.   Reports any hazards or faulty equipment to trained nurse.

7.3.   Following training it is the job holder's responsibility to ensure that she/he is fully conversant with Health and Safety Procedures and her/his role in emergency situations including; cardiac arrest procedures, fire procedures, infection control policy, lifting and handling policy and summoning security in the event of an incident occurring.

# 8. GENERAL

8.1.   It is implicit in this job description that the person be familiar with and adhere to all Trust and Directorate Policies and Guidelines within the sphere of responsibility.

8.2.   The job description will be subject to regular review and maybe amended in the light of demands of the unit.

**PERSON SPECIFICATION: Health care assistant. NVQ level 2/B Grade.**

| Essential | Desirable |
|---|---|
| Good basic education | Working towards or willing to undertake NVQ |
| Good communication skills Both written and verbal | |
| Able to use own initiative within guidelines. | |
| Able to work as part of a team and under the direction of qualified nurses. | |
| Experience of working with people | Previous experience in women's health |
| Adaptable, polite and reliable. | |
| Willing to adapt to change. | |
| Interest in women's health | |
| Ability to work a flexible shift pattern | |
| Punctual. | |

## Qualified nurses

The roles of qualified nurses in clinic vary considerably according to grade and experience. All clinics should have a minimum of one qualified nurse and one HCA. It is important to remember in light of the development of nurse practitioners that not all nurses wish to undertake new roles or responsibilities and that a clinic full of NP would not function without some staff undertaking a more traditional role.

Qualified nurses should be responsible for the management and smooth running of the clinic sessions. They should also be able to judge how long patients can expect to wait and inform patients accordingly. They should ensure, along with the HCA, that the rooms are prepared and should assist medical staff in examinations and procedures. Nursing staff will need to have or be able to find information for patients on all procedures and conditions that are seen within gynaecology. Qualified nurses are expected to act as advocates for patients and help them to make informed choices within the clinic. They also have to have experience to deal with any telephone queries and be able to pass these on to the relevant staff if they cannot resolve them. They should in conjunction with other nursing staff be responsible for ensuring that the clinic is kept well supplied. There will also need to be an experienced nurse who is the lead for the nursing staff; she/he may undertake the traditional role of the nurse within outpatients or a progressive role (see Job Descriptions E and F Grade Nurses).

### 1. JOB DETAILS

**JOB TITLE:**             Staff Nurse – Gynaecology

**GRADE:**             E

### 2. JOB PURPOSE

The gynaecology service aims to provide an integrated care. At present we have a core team of outpatient nurses and inpatient staff. This post is predominantly based within gynaecology outpatients with a specific remit for the development of nurse-led pre-operation assessment clinics. The role involves the responsibility for delivering and directing programmes of care, supervision of team members and co-ordination of the team and clinic areas in the absence of the team leader. The post holder also acts as a resource person for an area of practice related to women's health and will be supported to develop specialist knowledge in gynaecology. The post holder will also link with the dedicated pre-admission nurse for the day surgery unit to develop best practice and to provide cover if needed. The post holder is expected to rotate to the ward with specific learning objectives, if the needs of the service dictate.

KEY RESULT AREAS:

## 3. CLINICAL

3.1. Demonstrate clinical excellence within gynaecological nursing.
3.2. Promote partnership with women in the care process.
3.3. Work with team members to further develop clinical experience and strive to ensure that all nursing practice is based on sound rationale.
3.4. Work within and contribute to the running of the gynaecology outpatient services.
3.5. Assist in facilitating a therapeutic environment that meets the needs and wishes of the women.
3.6. Contribute actively to the ongoing development of the unit philosophy.
3.7. Recognize the importance of role model function.
3.8. Work with multidisciplinary team to ensure that all care is co-ordinated and investigation results are acted upon, liaising with the multidisciplinary team as appropriate
3.9. To develop and lead in conjunction with the outpatients team leader nurse-led pre-operation assessment clinic to facilitate a smooth admission process to the gynaecology ward.
3.10. To liaise with the admission staff and give a clinical input into the management of the waiting lists.
3.11. To liaise with the nurse undertaking pre-operation assessment clinics within day surgery and provide cover if necessarily.
3.12. Undertake a full and holistic assessment of women prior to operation, including any special needs in relation to discharge planning.
3.13. To provide women with full information in regard to their condition, operation and recovery.

## 4. EDUCATION

4.1. Accept personal responsibility for identifying own learning needs, professional development and updating, and take steps to pursue objectives.
4.2. Contribute to the development of teaching strategies to meet the need of staff and patients. Share new knowledge with team members.
4.3. Accept the roles of preceptor/mentor/assessor for junior staff, learners and NVQ candidates.
4.4. Assist in the facilitation of an environment, which is conducive to the acquisition of further knowledge and skills.
4.5. Accept responsibility as resource person in keeping the team updated in a relevant area.

## 5. MANAGEMENT

5.1. Take responsibility for the management of the clinic and patient care in the absence of senior staff with the aim of setting highest possible standards.

5.2. Act as a change agent to promote innovation and high practice standards.

5.3. Ensure the promotion of safety, well-being and interest of the women, staff and all visitors to the area.

5.4. Ensure that self and all staff adhere to all district and unit policies and procedures.

5.5. Contribute to monitoring the performance of junior staff .

5.6. Act as care co-ordinator for a dedicated group of patients.

5.7. Contribute to meeting the clinical objectives of the unit.

5.8. Contribute to development and evaluation of the unit standards.

## 6. AUDIT AND RESEARCH

6.1. Participate in the clinical audit activities within the unit.

6.2. Actively seek to improve practice through application of evidence.

6.3. Identify potential research areas within the Unit and propose study options.

6.4. Be receptive and supportive to the research plans of others.

## 7. GENERAL

7.1. It is implicit in this job description that the person be familiar with and adhere to all Trust and Directorate Policies and Guidelines within the sphere of responsibility.

7.2. The job description will be subject to regular review and maybe amended in the light of demands of the Unit.

7.3. The post holder will act at all times in accordance with the UKCC Code of Professional Conduct.

## PERSON SPECIFICATION: Named Nurse – Gynaecology

| Essential | Desirable |
|---|---|
| **Physical characteristics**<br>Can demonstrate good general health.<br>Is able to display a professional, presentation. | |
| **Qualifications**<br>Registered nurse<br>Willingness to undertake learning at diploma/degree level in an area related to women's health. | Counselling course.<br>Diploma/Degree level course in relevant field. |
| **Work experience**<br>Has previous experience in gynaecology, either ward or inpatient areas.<br>Can demonstrate experience of supervision of learners and trained staff.<br>Has proven experience of shift/clinic co-ordination ability. | Experience within surgery/oncology.<br>Supervision experience.<br>Previous experience of pre-clerking and outpatient support. |
| **Specialized knowledge**<br>Can show an awareness of the changing management of gynaecological care.<br>Can demonstrate an in-depth knowledge of and health promotion working knowledge in standard s etting and quality management. | |
| **Skills, abilities, attitudes, Motivation**<br>Can prove an ability to motivate others to promote ongoing development of gynaecology nursing.<br>Can demonstrate a commitment to teaching/sharing knowledge.<br>Can show a non-judgmental approach to care.<br>Can demonstrate effective communication skills.<br>Can prove a positive approach to change.<br>Can demonstrate evidence of motivation to keep up to date. | Can demonstrate ability to undertake intravenous drug administration.<br><br>Can demonstrate phlebotomy and venous cannulation skills.<br><br>Can prove a basic computer literacy in Windows and hospital systems. |
| **Special aptitudes**<br>Shows an enthusiasm towards teaching/ sharing knowledge. | Can prove an up to date professional profile. |
| **Circumstances**<br>Can show an able to work flexible hours to meet service need. | |

## 1. JOB DETAILS

JOB TITLE:                    Team Leader – Gynaecology Outpatients

GRADE:                        F

## 2. JOB PURPOSE

Working as a team leader the post holder has in-depth knowledge of gynaecology nursing and uses this to deliver and co-ordinate high standards of practice.

The post holder will ensure the effective day-to-day management of the gynaecology outpatients department.

The post holder should work in conjunction with the nurse practitioner to develop new services within outpatients

## KEY RESPONSIBILITIES

## 3. CLINICAL

3.1 Assess, plan, implement and evaluate care to meet women's individual needs within the outpatient setting.

3.2 Set and evaluate standards of care; supervise and teach other nursing and non-nursing staff.

3.3 Co-ordinate the clinics on a daily basis. Liaising with clerical and medical staff to avoid problems.

3.4 Undertakes management duties within the clinic setting, e.g. the management of staff, rostering staff.

3.5 Determine nursing priorities and with minimal guidance deliver skilled practical nursing care.

3.6 Deliver nursing care within the changing demands of the unit.

3.7 To develop nurse-led pre-admission clinics.

3.8 To develop and run other nurse led clinics, e.g. post operative follow-up insertion of ring pessaries.

3.9 To participate in the running of one-stop minor procedures clinics.

3.10 To act as a chaperone and advocate for women in the clinics.

3.11 Participate in the care, custody and administration of medicines in accordance with the Trust policy.

3.12 Take responsibility for ensuring safe moving and handling techniques.

3.13 Work with other team members to ensure that all care is co-ordinated and investigation results are acted upon, liaising with the multidisciplinary team as appropriate

3.14 To ensure that infection control guidelines are followed within the outpatients.

3.15 To be the link from outpatients to the directorate Health and Safety group.

## 4. PROFESSIONAL

4.1  Ensure that all clinical and legal documents completed are both accurate and legible and that nurses understand their relevance and the confidentiality of their nature.

4.2  Assist in maintaining accurate collection of patient activity data.

4.3  To participate in the development and use of electronic patient records.

4.4  Take personal responsibility for own professional development and keep up to date with developments and research.

## 5. EDUCATIONAL

5.1  Participate in the Unit teaching programme.

5.2  Contribute to the development of teaching strategies to meet the needs of staff and patients. Share new knowledge with team members.

5.3  Accept the roles of preceptor/mentor/assessor to ensure skill development and evaluation of junior staff, learners and NVQ candidates.

5.4  Accept responsibility as resource person in keeping the team updated in a relevant area.

5.5  Ensure that learners allocated to the department are given appropriate teaching, support and guidance in accordance with ward objectives and continuous assessment.

## 6. MANAGEMENT

6.1  Act as a change agent to promote innovation and high practice standards.

6.2  Inform Senior Nurse of incidents/conditions, which affect standards of care. Participate in the risk management of the unit.

6.3  Ensure effective communications with all disciplines, patients and families.

6.4  Participate in ordering supplies as required within the agreed budget.

6.5  Ensure resources are used carefully and wastage avoided.

6.6  To participate in the staff management of the outpatient setting, including appraisals, performance management, disciplinary, rota and covering of clinics where appropriate.

## 7. AUDIT AND RESEARCH

7.1  Participate in the clinical audit activities within the Unit.

7.2  Actively seek to improve practice through application of evidence.

7.3  Identify potential research areas within the Unit and propose study options.

7.4  Be receptive and supportive to the research plans of others.

## 8. GENERAL

8.1 The post holder is expected to be familiar with and adhere to all Trust and Directorate Policies and Guidelines within the sphere of responsibility.

8.2 The job description will be subject to regular review and may be amended in the light of demands of the unit.

8.3 The post holder will act at all times in accordance with the UKCC Code of Professional Conduct.

### PERSON SPECIFICATION: Team Leader, Gynaecology, Grade F

| Essential | Desirable |
|---|---|
| Registered nurse with at least 2 years' experience in gynaecology/women's health nursing, and at least 12 months' experience at E grade. | Counselling course. |
| To have obtained or be working towards either the ENB225 or a Women's Health Diploma/Degree. Willingness to undertake further study and to develop practice | ENB 998, 901, 931 or other relevant ENB course Experience in outpatient setting desirable. |
| *Can demonstrate phlebotomy and venous cannulation skills or willingness to undertake training* | Is able to insert speculums and take swabs and smears. |
| Able to assess, plan, implement, evaluate and prioritise patient care without supervision | Experience within surgery / oncology, and within outpatients setting and of pre-clerking. |
| Displays a non-judgmental approach to care. | Preceptor to qualified staff. |
| Experience of standard setting and quality management. | Experience of oncology/bereavement care. |
| Has proven experience of shift co-ordination. | Can prove a basic computer literacy in Windows and hospital systems. |
| Ability to prioritise own workload | |
| Can show an awareness of the changing management of gynaecology care and has a positive approach to change. | |
| Can demonstrate ability to undertake intra-venous drug administration. | |
| Can demonstrate knowledge of relevant health and safety issues | |
| Demonstrate ability to work within the multidisciplinary team | |
| Demonstrates effective verbal and written communication skills. | |
| Evidence of ongoing professional development | |
| Can demonstrate experience of supervision and teaching of learners and trained staff. | |
| Demonstrates a commitment to teaching/sharing knowledge. | |
| Can show knowledge of current trends in Women's Health | |
| Demonstrate awareness of budgetary and resource management. | |
| Knowledge of audit and evidence based practice and willingness to participate in audit and research | |

## Nurse practitioners (NP)

The traditional role of the nurse within clinics has been limited to chaperoning and assisting, explanation and advice, and the follow-up of results. Nursing staff are now more frequently undertaking new roles and learning new skills. Nurses who undertake a new role are frequently called nurse practitioners or clinical nurse specialists. As expectations and health care changes nurses are the front-line staff and need to be innovative in creating new ways to answer the needs of their patients.

Many pre-admission clinics are now entirely undertaken by nursing staff that have received additional training in physical examinations and history taking skills and will liase directly with the patient's consultant if there are any problems. Nurses of any grade can decide to extend their skills and role, of paramount importance in this is that they have had additional training and education to carry out this role and have support from all staff to do so. Other examples for an extended nursing role can be seen in relation to continence care, zoladex and HRT implants. Nurses who have a particular interest may only work as a nurse practitioner in certain clinics and then revert to a more traditional role for others. Owing to the large number of sub-specialities in gynaecology this chapter will not describe the training required for NPs in detail as it has been included in some relevant chapters and needs to be discussed and agreed locally.

A NP works at an advanced clinical level, which includes providing expert practice, undertaking holistic consultations, critical thinking and utilization of decision-making skills, leadership, and education and service development. The NP can work in a multidisciplinary team in some clinics and then in a nurse-led team for other services.

Generally NPs will have had a long career in gynaecology nursing in a variety of different settings. This is important in ensuring that they have the correct knowledge but also in establishing clinical credibility within the medical and nursing teams.

As well as having practical skills the NP needs to have undertaken further educational qualifications in order to obtain the theoretical underpinnings to her practice.

In developing NPs in all sub-specialities of gynaecology it is essential that training ensures:

1.  That the NP is able to recognize normal and abnormal anatomy and physiology.
2.  That the NP is confidently, competently and safely able to take the history and perform intimate examinations.
3.  That their management plans are in line with national and local guidelines and protocols.
4.  That the NP is aware of the legalities associated with the role extension and her professional practice.

# JOB DETAILS

**1. JOB TITLE:**          Nurse Practitioner – Gynaecology outpatients

**GRADE:**              G Grade

## 2. JOB PURPOSE

With an in-depth knowledge of gynaecological nursing practice, the post holder acts as a nurse practitioner and expert in the area of gynaecological care within outpatient services. The post holder will work in conjunction with the nurse consultant for outpatients to ensure that the highest quality of evidenced-based care is delivered to women. As a senior team member this post holds key responsibility for communication and team leadership across the Unit.

The post holder will act autonomously, having a primary responsibility for developing a specialist/practitioner focus within gynaecology. The practitioner will facilitate effective communication links with both the Primary Healthcare and Trust multidisciplinary teams. The post holder will act as a lead for Clinical Governance and risk management within the outpatients department.

The post holder will develop and facilitate nurse practice across the speciality of gynaecology liaising with other nurse specialist nurses. This post will have specific responsibility for leading interdisciplinary teams within the outpatient settings and for the strategic management of the nurse role.

The post holder will also have a role working with the admissions team to ensure that the management of the waiting list has a clinical focus and is managed tin accordance with DOH and Trust initiatives.

The post holder will participate in the collaborative management of the Gynaecology Unit.

## KEY RESPONSIBILITIES

### 1. CLINICAL

1.1. To demonstrate clinical excellence within gynaecological nursing.
1.2. To promote partnership with women in the care process.
1.3. To demonstrate a commitment to advancing nursing practice by research.
1.4. To ensure evidence-based nursing practice.
1.5. To develop skills in history taking, critical decision making, patient examination, pre-assessment clinics and nurse discharge.
1.6. To act as clinical supervisor to an identified peer group.
1.7. To promote and develop the outpatient service in conjunction with the multidisciplinary team.

1.8. To establish links with other provider units to aid dissemination of information and best practice.

1.9. To develop a therapeutic environment that meets the needs and wishes of the women.

1.10. To, in partnership with the multi disciplinary team, take the lead to coordinate the development of protocols and guidelines.

## 2. EDUCATIONAL

2.1. To provide leadership to team members, encouraging and directing innovation and ongoing nursing development.

2.2. To teach, both formally and informally, within the Gynaecology Unit.

2.3. To accept personal responsibility for keeping up-to-date and identifying own learning needs.

2.4. To act as an effective role model and mentor in the demonstration of high standards of practice.

2.5. To act as an assessor/supervisor for junior staff, learners and NVQ candidates.

2.6. To promote continual professional development in all staff.

2.7. To regularly take part in the multi disciplinary meetings within gynaecology.

## 3. MANAGEMENT

3.1. To be aware of resource implications and aim for a cost effective care delivery.

3.2. To act as a change agent to promote innovation and high practice standards.

3.3. To ensure team commitment to the Unit, Trust and Government directives, e.g. 'Patients charter'.

3.4. To be responsible for the collation of comments and complaints within the Outpatient settings and formulate action plans to address identified issues.

3.5. To ensure promotion of well being, safety and interests of the women, staff, and visitors to the clinical area.

3.6. To ensure maintenance of nursing and clinical records in accordance with current guidelines.

3.7. To monitor and appraise performance of junior staff.

3.8. To collect activity data and statistics as requested by the Women's services management team.

3.9. To be fully conversant with Health and Safety Procedures and report any accidents/hazards to the appropriate department.

3.10. To act as the outpatients department's lead in clinical Governance and risk management.

# 4. AUDIT AND RESEARCH

4.1.  To participate in the clinical audit activities within the unit.

4.2.  To actively seek to improve practice through application of research.

4.3.  To identify potential research areas within the unit and propose study options.

4.4.  To identify own research projects as identified with the Clinical Nurse Manager.

4.5.  To contribute to the research plans of others.

# 5. GENERAL

5.1.  It is implicit in this job description that the person be familiar with and adhere to all Trust and Directorate policies and guidelines within the sphere of responsibility.

5.2.  The job description will be subject to regular review and maybe amended in the light of demands of the unit.

5.3.  The post holder will act at all times in accordance with the NMC Code of Professional Conduct.

## PERSON SPECIFICATION: Nurse Practitioner – Gynaecology G Grade

| Essential | Desirable | Means of assessment |
|---|---|---|
| **Clinical** | | |
| Minimum of 12 months experience at F grade in acute gynaecology/outpatients. Substantial experience in gynaecology. In depth knowledge of gynaecology outpatients. Previous related experience. Previous experience of smear, high vaginal swab taking and pelvic examination skills. Phlebotomy and venous cannulation skills. | Previous experience in practitioner role. Skilled in assessment of need and insertion of hormone replacement implants. Skilled at insertion of vaginal pessaries. | Interview/ documentation |
| **Educational** | | |
| Registered nurse Women's Health Diploma/ENB 225/be willing to undertake studies at advanced level ENB 998. Degree level course in relevant field or willing to undertake course. Evidence of motivation to keep up-to-date. | Relevant women's health courses. Counselling course. Certificate in Ultrasound scanning. Budget management. | Documentation |
| **Management** | | |
| Awareness of the changing management of gynaecology. Can demonstrate knowledge of current trends in women's health. Ability to motivate others to promote ongoing development of gynaecology nursing. | Clinical supervision experience. Supervision of trained staff. Experience of developing protocols. | Interview Test References |

Committed to teaching/sharing knowledge.
Can demonstrate and awareness of Clinical
Governance.
Effective communication skills.
Skills in diplomacy.
Demonstrated evidence of leadership skills.
Supervision of learners.

**Audit and research**

| | | |
|---|---|---|
| Working knowledge in standard setting and quality management. Knowledge of risk management. Experience of participating in audit. | Project management experience. Has undertaken own research or audit. | Interview |

**General**

| | | |
|---|---|---|
| Positive approach to change. Computer literacy in Windows and hospital systems. Enthusiastic. Able to work calmly in pressured environments. Able to act as the women's advocate. Able to work flexible hours to meet the needs of the service. | | References /interview |

## 1. JOB DETAILS

**JOB TITLE:**          Senior Nurse Practitioner – Colposcopy Services

**GRADE:**          G/H Grade

## 2. JOB PURPOSE

With an in-depth knowledge of gynaecology and health promotion the senior nurse is responsible for the co-ordination of all activities within the Colposcopy service. The post holder leads a team of nurses, clinicians and administrative staff and is responsible for the co-ordination of the programmes of care management for all the complete caseload. The post holder is identified as the lead clinician and works in partnership with a named Consultant to deliver clinical objectives for the Colposcopy service. The post holder is identified as having financial management responsibility to deliver the service within the agreed budget.

As an accredited Colposcopist the post holder acts as an autonomous practitioner in undertaking diagnostic and therapeutic clinic sessions, taking responsibility and accountability for appropriate clinical management and care programmes. The post holder is responsible for the standards of training and supervision within the unit for medical and nursing staff.

The Colposcopy Unit is part of the Gynaecology Directorate with its aim of delivery of an integrated care for women. The postholder participates in the collaborative management of the Gynaecology Unit, is recognized as a key member of the Management Team and is expected to act up in the absence of the Clinical Nurse Manager.

## 3. CLINICAL RESPONSIBILITIES

3.1. Demonstrate clinical excellence within gynaecological nursing, specifically colposcopy.

3.2. Maintain clinical credibility through demonstration of own ongoing professional learning and expert role model practice.

3.3. Undertake own diagnostic and treatment sessions and care programmes within defined boundaries.

3.4. Ensure an evidence-based clinical practice.

3.5. Develop methods for delivering, evaluating and continuously monitoring clinical care.

3.6. Act as clinical supervisor to an identified peer group.

3.7. Demonstrate a commitment to advancing nursing practice by research and evidence.

3.8. Establish links with other provider units to aid dissemination of information and best practice.

3.9. Continually review and update information to meet the changing needs and expectations of clients.

3.10. Develop a therapeutic environment that meets the needs and wishes of the women.

## 4. MANAGEMENT

4.1. Co-ordinate the care and follow-up management for a defined client group.

4.2. Effectively manage the non-pay budget for the Colposcopy Unit. Be aware of resource implications and aim for a cost effective care delivery.

4.3. Ensure appropriate use of staff resources to enable a safe, efficient and reliable service.

4.4. Ensure adherence to fail safe standards and processes.

4.5. Ensure promotion of well-being, safety and interests of patients, staff and visitors to the Unit.

4.6. Act as a change agent to promote innovation and high practice standards.

4.7. Ensure team commitment to the Unit, Trust and Government directives.

4.8. Be responsible for the response to complaints and collation of comments, formulating action plans to address identified issues.

4.9. Ensure maintenance of nursing and clinical records in accordance with current guidelines.

4.10. Monitor and appraise performance of junior staff.

4.11. Participate in the recruitment and selection of nursing staff across the Gynaecology Unit.

4.12. Collect activity data and statistics as requested by the Gynaecology Management Team.

4.13. Be fully conversant with Health and Safety Procedures, take responsibility for management and report any accidents/hazards to the appropriate department.

## 5. EDUCATIONAL

5.1. Provide leadership to team members, encouraging and directing innovation and ongoing clinical development.

5.2. Teach both formally and informally, within the Gynaecology Unit.

5.3. Identify development and learning needs with junior staff and work with Team Leaders to provide strategies and opportunities to address those needs.

5.4. Accept personal responsibility for keeping up-to-date and identifying own learning needs.

5.5. Undertake updating and development required to maintain accreditation as nurse colposcopist.

5.6. Act as an effective role model and mentor in the demonstration of high standards of practice.

5.7. Act as an assessor/supervisor for junior staff, learners and NVQ candidates.

5.8. Promote continual professional development in all staff.

5.9. Facilitate a learning environment conducive to the acquisition of further knowledge and skills.

## 6. AUDIT AND RESEARCH

6.1. Participate in the clinical audit activities within the unit.

6.2. Undertake yearly audit of own clinical colposcopy activity.

6.3. Actively seek to improve practice through application of research.

6.4. Identify potential research areas within the Unit and propose study options.

6.5. Identify own research projects as identified with the Clinical Nurse Manager.

6.6. Contribute to the research plans of others.

## 7. GENERAL

7.1. It is implicit in this job description that the person be familiar with and adhere to all Trust and Directorate policies and guidelines within the sphere of responsibility.

7.2. The job description will be subject to regular review and maybe amended in the light of demands of the unit.

7.3. The post holder will be required to act up for the Clinical Nurse Manager as appropriate and participate in management cover with other senior team leaders.

7.4. The post holder will act at all times in accordance with the UKCC Code of Professional Conduct.

## PERSON SPECIFICATION: Senior Nurse/Practitioner – Colposcopy Services

| Essential | Desirable |
|---|---|
| Registered nurse<br>BSCCP accredited Nurse Colposcopist.<br>Degree in nursing/health studies.<br>Women's Health Diploma/ENB 225 or equivalent and be willing to undertake studies at advanced level. | ENB 998/Teaching certificate.<br>Degree level course in relevant field.<br>Counselling Course<br>Family Planning/Practice Nurse certificates. |
| Able to demonstrate experiential learning from three and half years experience in gynaecology/women's health. | Clinical supervision experience.<br>2 years F Grade experience.<br>Previous experience in practitioner role. |
| Proven experience in supervision of learners.<br>Proven experience in supervision of trained staff.<br>Able to show evidence of teaching and practice development in others.<br>Able to demonstrate ward and team management and previous leadership role.<br>Able to demonstrate proven project management experience. | Budget management. |
| Able to demonstrate an awareness of the changing management of diagnostic and therapeutic colposcopy.<br>Able to demonstrate a working knowledge in standard setting and quality management | |
| Proven ability to motivate others to promote ongoing development of gynaecology nursing.<br>Committed to teaching/sharing knowledge.<br>Demonstrates a non-judgmental approach to care.<br>Developed skills in pelvic examination, smear and high vaginal smear taking.<br>Developed phlebotomy and venous cannulation skills.<br>Demonstrates effective communication skills.<br>Shows a positive approach to change.<br>Demonstrates a basic computer literacy.<br>Evidence of motivation to keep up to date. | Advanced assessment skills.<br><br>Computer literacy in Windows and hospital systems. |
| Proven enthusiasm towards teaching/sharing knowledge.<br>Can show an up to date professional profile. | |
| Enthusiastic.<br>Approachable and friendly.<br>Able to recognize stress in self and others. | |
| Able to work flexible hours to meet service need. | |

## Nurse consultants

The National Plan has outlined a role for nurse consultants. Gynaecology outpatients is one area that they could be employed. A nurse consultant is expected to undertake her own caseload of patients and be an expert in nursing for that area. As the care of women with gynaecology problems is changing and many more patients are being managed on a medical outpatient basis this can give rise to the nurse consultant. There are many areas in gynaecology that would lend themselves to nurse consultants:

- colposcopy;
- one-stop clinics;
- menstrual dysfunction;
- menopause.

A nurse consultant needs to have a minimum of a master's level education and the additional skills required will depend on the specific remit of the role. It is also written into the job that the nurse must spend at least 50% of her/his time in education and research. This it is hoped can only serve to further nurses' education in the outpatient setting and nursing research related to gynaecology. The job description for a nurse in bleeding/menstrual dysfunction is shown in detail in Job Description Nurse Consultant, as an example of how consultant nurses can work and the training requirements needed.

The nurse consultant role that is proposed here is within the outpatient service and carries a specific caseload for the menstrual dysfunction/one-stop clinics. These clinics are particularly useful for women with abnormal vaginal bleeding, cervical polyps or skin disorders of the vulva that require a biopsy

Out of the 10 000 referrals that are received by the outpatients clinic each year. Referrals that fit into the above categories now represent one quarter of the total referrals to the outpatients department. At present nurses play a very minor role in the care of these women and it is proposed that the nurse consultant will carry this caseload and promote nursing practice, health promotion and aim to improve the quality of life for the patients within this single clinic visit. With the reorganization of the workforce and the introduction of a nurse consultant the care will become more efficient and a seamless and integrated service be provided.

### Nurse consultant in bleeding/menstrual dysfunction

The post holder will lead the care within the one-stop menstrual dysfunction/minor procedures clinic.

**Clinical practice.** There is much scope and demand within gynaecology outpatient services to improve nursing knowledge and critical decision making as well as increasing the scope of nursing practice.

Traditionally gynaecology outpatient nursing is seen as an area where the only input nurses have is as chaperones. With the changes in technology and advancing of medicine there is more scope for the input of nurses into the case management of patients.

The post holder will be an expert in menstrual dysfunction and bleeding problems including the menopause and specifically management on an outpatient basis. The management and care of these women requiring one clinic visit and follow-up consultations via phone if necessary, will improve the care of these women and ensure continuity.

The post holder will be an equal member of the multi-professional consultant team within the women's health directorate.

**Education.** The post holder will be a practising nurse with a minimum of a master's level education. In addition to this she/he should possess post basis courses in women's health.

The post holder will identify development and training needs within the outpatient service. She will be instrumental in the development of training packages to extend the role and scope of nursing within the department.

The post holder would also be expected to be responsible for the education of other professional staff in relation to menstrual dysfunction.

**Research and development.** The nursing care of women in gynaecology outpatients is particularly under researched, with most research concentrating on medical treatments. The post holder would be expected to promote nursing research within the unit as well as conducting research into nursing practice within the gynaecology outpatients.

The post holder would also be expected to assist all staff in the development and reviewing of protocols that are relevant to nursing and the department.

**Management.** The post holder will contribute to the clinical management within the outpatient setting. Women requiring appointments for menstrual dysfunction will be seen by the nurse consultant. This will involve one member of staff streamlining care and making decisions. The development of this service will lead to improved nursing care, shorter waiting times for patients for first appointments and continuity of care. With the introduction of this post there will be a knock on effect to the whole directorate. There will be fewer women being referred to the day surgery list for simple procedures, which will free up spaces for the more complex laparoscopy work.

**Job plan.** The post holder will be involved in clinical care for 50% of the working week. This will be five clinical sessions, four of these in direct patient contact and one involved with the telephone helpline. She will be based in the gynaecology outpatients department. The remaining 50% of the time she will be involved in identifying; setting up and conditioning research into nursing care and one stop clinics. She will also be expected to teach junior staff within the unit. It is expected that the post holder will contribute to the ongoing philosophy of inter professional working and education within the department.

## 1. JOB DETAILS

JOB TITLE: Consultant nurse – menstrual dysfunction/One-stop clinics

## 2. JOB PURPOSE

This post is based in the women's service gynaecology outpatients' department. This is open Monday to Friday from 8.30 to 6.00 p.m. and has nine clinic sessions each week. The department receives referrals internally, from GP's. The post holder will be responsible for seeing women that have simple menstrual dysfunction, especially within the one-stop see and treat clinics. The post holder will provide consultation and advice for professionals in the assessment, management and treatment of menstrual disorders.

Responsibility will include the furthering of nursing practice, research and care within this area of expertise.

The post holder will have extensive theoretical and practical knowledge and experience of the clinical skills that would be needed within modern gynaecology outpatients.

The post holder will act as a clinical lead for women attending the menstrual dysfunction clinics.

## KEY RESPONSIBILITIES

## 1. CLINICAL PRACTICE

1.1. To use advanced nursing skills to assess the physical and psychosocial needs of the patients within the caseload.
1.2. Provide evidence based information to patients to facilitate informed choices.
1.3. To determine in partnership with the patients the most appropriate management and treatment plan.
1.4. Take a clinical responsibility for women attending the one-stop menstrual dysfunction clinics and menopause service.
1.5 Act as an advocate for the women under your care.
1.6. To become an independent prescriber in relation to clinical area.

## 2. PROFESSIONAL LEADERSHIP

2.1.  Act as a consultant to nurses and other staff in the unit in relation to the area defined.
2.2.  To contribute to health improvement plans.
2.3.  Increase access to services by promoting and developing nurse led services.
2.4.  To work collaboratively and in partnership with practitioners from other disciplines and across organisational boundaries.
2.5.  To establish collaborative partnerships with primary care to encourage joint working and seamless care for patients, in person, via phone or email.
2.6.  Participate in and lead the development of the gynaecology nursing.

## 3. EDUCATION, TRAINING AND DEVELOPMENT

3.1.  To tutor and mentor nurse undertaking women's health courses and further studies within the directorate.
3.2.  Provide clinical teaching, support and guidance to nurses, students and medical staff.
3.3.  Identify developmental needs within the staff in outpatients and develop these staff to extend the role of the nurse.
3.4.  To provide education and training informally and through formal courses.
3.5.  To provide tuition in practical skills.

## 4. PRACTICE AND SERVICE DEVELOPMENT, RESEARCH AND EVALUATION

4.1.  To review the evidence base for clinical practice within this field and to disseminate information and evidence that will lead to the improvement of knowledge, treatment and management options.
4.2.  To review the service and implement improvements in line with progressive practice and research evidence.
4.3.  To develop standards and guideline for assessment, management and treatment of menstrual disorders.
4.4.  To lead or participate in and facilitate others in the conducting of research aimed at improving care.
4.5.  To conduct and support audit.

# PERSON SPECIFICATION: Consultant nurse – menstrual dysfunction – One-stop clinics

| Essential | Desirable |
|---|---|
| **Education** | |
| | Ultrasound scanning course |
| RGN | Counselling course |
| Educated to MSc or above | Evidence of further education in research |
| ENB higher award in gynaecology | or audit |
| Nursing | ENB 901/family planning course |
| ENB 998 | PhD in health related studies |
| **Professional** | |
| Proven professional development | |
| Can demonstrate professional accountability | |
| Ability to demonstrate a thorough | |
| understanding of recent Government papers. | |
| **Skills and attributes** | |
| Good communication skills | Ultrasound scanning experience |
| Ability to work autonomously while | Advanced practical skills |
| being part of a team | Counselling skills |
| Proven critical decision making skills | Previous experience of change management |
| Interpersonal skills | |
| Presentation skills | |
| Proven training and teaching ability | |
| Motivation | |
| Computer literate | |
| Previous leadership role | |
| **Experience** | |
| Extensive practice at a senior level within | Extensive practice within all areas of |
| gynaecology | gynaecology |
| Experience of working as a nurse | Publication of own research |
| practitioner showing ability to work at an | Previous management role |
| advanced level. | Previous experience as mentor/preceptor |
| Proven and established expertise in | |
| gynaecology | |
| Previous experience of working with students | |
| Previous knowledge of research and audit | |
| Experience of writing reviewing | |
| guidelines/protocols | |
| Knowledge and use of computers in healthcare | |
| **Personal qualities** | |
| Reliable and punctual | |
| Academically orientated | |
| Research orientated | |
| Assertive | |
| Organized | |
| Innovative | |

Specialist registrars and second/third year SHOs who are new to the department should be allowed to see patients independently but for the first few weeks they should come and discuss every case with the consultant. This has several benefits. It allows the consultant to assess the ability of the junior doctor to evaluate a case, develop a management plan, justify their management plan and their communication abilities. It also allows the consultant to know about the cases going through the clinic. Junior medical staff are often very up to date in their knowledge because they are preparing for postgraduate examinations. The consultant should be open to learning from the junior staff in the same way that junior staff expect to learn from consultants. The junior staff may find the application of their knowledge more difficult and this is where the consultant can help. If the consultant is unapproachable or the clinic is overbooked then this healthy learning relationship cannot work and the patient is left exposed to the vagaries in the knowledge and ability of the junior doctor.

Junior doctors should dictate their letters during the clinic and for the first few weeks these should be checked by the consultant before being sent. This is another teaching opportunity to improve standards.

# Index

WITHDRAWN